Intermittent Fasting for Women

The Effortless Guide for Beginners to Lose Weight, Burn Fat and Heal Your Body

Written by

CHERYL CARRIER

TABLE OF CONTENTS

Introduction

Intermittent fasting is now a trend among those who want to lose weight. If you are concerned about your weight and want to lose excess fats, then maybe it is time to give intermittent fasting a try. Women who are greatly concerned about improving their figure and physique can also choose to implement intermittent fasting. However, it is crucial to understand how this eating pattern works before beginning to follow it.

If you are one of those women aiming to lose weight through IF, then you have to research how it works and gather other information that will guide you in making it work in your favor. By increasing your knowledge about intermittent fasting for women, you will be able to understand how to make it work.

Your acquired knowledge about this eating pattern will be useful in making the right decisions. You will know exactly how you can maximize its benefits. With the help of this book, you will get an idea of what intermittent fasting is. You will be guided in making this eating pattern a part of your life and ensuring that you gain all its positive effects as far as your health and fitness are concerned.

Chapter 1 – Intermittent Fasting and How Does it Work?

Intermittent fasting is a famous eating pattern practiced by those who would like to lose weight and improve their health. It is not a diet plan, though. It is an eating pattern, which involves putting your meals on schedule. You schedule your meals in a way that you can maximize their positive effects on your body.

If you want to try intermittent fasting for women, then note that it does not require you to change what you eat. What you will be changing is when or the exact time you eat. Many women consider IF as a great approach for losing weight. It is also an effective way of becoming lean without dramatically cutting down calories or following a crazy diet.

Intermittent fasting even allows you to still eat the same amount of calories as before, although you have to do so during your eating window. It is an effective approach to maintaining your muscle mass while also becoming lean. Aside from that, many go for this approach because of convenience. It lets you get rid of excess weight while only requiring you to make minor behavioral changes.

How Does Intermittent Fasting Work?

Intermittent fasting works by alternating certain periods of being in the fed and fasted state. You can do this eating pattern in different ways – among which are alternate-day fasting and meal skipping.

One term you have to be aware of if you want to try IF is the fed state.

It is the specific time when your body digests and absorbs food. It starts once you begin to eat. In most cases, the fed state lasts for around 3-5 hours while your body absorbs and digests what you have consumed. During your fed state, your body may have a hard time doing the fat-burning process since you will have high levels of insulin during this period.

Once the fed state is done, the post-absorptive state comes next. It lasts for around 8 to 12 hours from the last meal you have consumed, the specific time when you go to the fasted state. During this state, you can expect your body to have an easier time burning fats due to your low insulin levels.

This is also the time when your body is capable of burning those fats that it can't access while you were still at the fed state. This state tends to burn fat effectively in the sense that you can lose excess fats without making drastic changes in the way you eat, the frequency of your exercise, and the amount of food you take in.

The good thing about intermittent fasting is that it does not only focus on helping you lose weight. It also provides other positive effects, like regulating your blood glucose, making your muscles lean, preventing coronary heart disease, and controlling your blood lipids.

Does Intermittent Fasting Work for Women?

Yes, it does. However, you have to familiarize yourself with the ins and outs of this eating pattern to make it truly work in your favor. Remember that a woman's body may have a different response to IF compared to that of men. It is more advisable for women to modify their intermittent fasting approach to fit their physique.

One thing that you can do, in this case, is to have shorter fasting periods as well as fewer fasting days. That way, you can gain as many benefits that men get from this eating pattern. You need to modify the approach since female bodies are often sensitive to restrictions in terms of calorie intake.

If you take in an extremely low amount of calories due to too long and frequent fasting periods, then it is greatly possible for the hypothalamus, a tiny part of your brain, to get drastically affected. It might hamper the secretion of hormone needed in releasing a couple of relaxing hormones – the follicle-stimulating hormones or FSH and the luteinizing hormone or LH.

The problem is that the inability of these hormones to communicate properly with your ovaries might lead to negative effects, like infertility, irregular periods, and poor bone health. To avoid those issues, you have to understand everything about intermittent fasting and how you can make it work for women. As mentioned, modifying your approach to this eating pattern can work wonders in achieving your desired results.

Chapter 2 – Benefits and Drawbacks of Intermittent Fasting for Women

It is important to note that intermittent fasting has its own share of benefits and drawbacks. Learn about such pros and cons so you can weigh them and decide whether it is safe for you to make this eating pattern a part of your life.

Health Benefits of Intermittent Fasting (Pros)

So what are the positive effects of intermittent fasting to a woman's health and body? Here are just a few of them that encourage most people to try out this eating pattern.

Promotes weight loss

One of the primary reasons why a lot of women try IF is to help them lose weight. It is not surprising as this eating pattern seems to be working well in that area. Through scheduled periods of eating and fasting, you can encourage yourself to eat fewer calories and meals. You can achieve that benefit, provided you do not compensate fasting period by eating excessively once your fed state comes in.

Apart from helping you take in fewer calories, intermittent fasting also improves the way your hormones function. It is a big help in facilitating weight loss. Sticking to this eating pattern makes it possible for you to increase your growth hormones and norepinephrine or noradrenaline as well as lower your insulin level. All these effects of IF aid in breaking down excess body fats and ensuring that they get used to increase your energy.

It is also the reason why even short-term fasting can boost your metabolism by around 3 to 14%. This is beneficial as it improves the ability of your body to burn more calories. IF is also an effective weight loss solution as it works in lowering your waist circumference. It means it plays a major role in getting rid of belly fat. Furthermore, it prevents you from losing too much muscle mass without restricting your calorie intake too much.

Improves your insulin sensitivity

Another great advantage of IF for women is that it helps in improving your insulin sensitivity and lowering your blood sugar sensitivity. Expect it to contribute to reducing your insulin resistance, which is a great advantage if you are prone to suffering from Type 2 diabetes or already suffering from it. By sticking to this eating pattern, you will most likely experience a reduction of 3% to 6% in your fasting blood sugar and 20% to 31% in your fasting insulin.

Reduces cholesterol

Probably one thing that makes intermittent fasting so effective in losing excess weight is that it usually requires you to eat during daytime – the specific period when your body has a natural desire to take in calories. It allows you to eat based on your circadian rhythm, which basically means consuming energy during your active hours then lowering your food intake at night when your body is no longer that active.

If you follow that rhythm, then your body will be able to do a more effective job in metabolizing your food better. It can lead to improved blood sugar as well as lipids, like triglycerides and cholesterol. With that in mind, it is safe to say that IF does a pretty good job of lowering your cholesterol.

This specific benefit is even more noticeable if you stick to the 5:2 intermittent fasting method, which we will discuss in the next chapter. With the 5:2 fasting method, you can lower your cholesterol as well as your risk of developing any heart disease.

Improves brain function

You will also be glad to know that intermittent fasting works in improving the way your brain functions. It contributes to improving a wide range of metabolic features that are necessary for promoting superior brain health.

One of these is reducing inflammation, oxidative stress, insulin resistance, and blood sugar. This famous eating pattern can also promote new nerve cell growth, which plays a huge role in boosting your brain function. Aside from that, it can raise your brain-derived neurotrophic factor or BDNF, which is an important brain hormone.

Note that the lack of this brain hormone can lead to depression and other brain issues, so it is necessary to have a good supply of it. Moreover, IF keeps your brain protected from the potential damage brought on by a stroke.

Positively changes the way your cells, hormones, and genes function

Through fasting or not eating for a while, you can expect a few changes in your body. One of these is initiating vital cell repair processes and making some changes in the level of your hormones, particularly those that help improve the accessibility of some stored body fats.

Intermittent fasting can facilitate some of these positive changes by improving the functions of your cells, hormones, and genes. It aids in reducing your level of insulin, which promotes fat burning. It can also significantly increase the level of human growth hormone (HGH), which is a good thing as it also contributes to effective muscle gain and fat burning.

Your body can also greatly benefit from the cellular repair processes that it can now efficiently perform, like getting rid of wastes from your cells. Aside from that, IF supports several beneficial changes in molecules and genes linked to increasing your lifespan and protecting you from various diseases.

Prevents inflammation and oxidative stress

One of the most common problems you have to avoid is oxidative stress as it might bring you closer towards experiencing premature signs of aging as well as dealing with chronic diseases. Oxidative stress makes use of free radicals, the unstable molecules that react with vital molecules in your body, such as DNA and protein, then cause damages to them.

Through intermittent fasting, you can protect yourself from the negative effects of oxidative stress. In addition, it can contribute to fighting inflammation, which can result in a wide range of common illnesses.

Improves skin health

Every woman wants to have clear and glowing skin, and that is what you can get from following intermittent fasting. Keep in mind that the foods you eat can directly affect the health of your skin as well as the way it looks. Certain unhealthy foods, like sugary beverages and snacks, can have a negative effect on your skin by causing your blood sugar to spike dramatically.

One skin issue that you might experience because of the food you eat is acne. Apart from foods, factors like high insulin level, lack of sleep, and inflammation can also cause your skin to age and become unhealthy. Since IF seems to tackle such issues well, it may serve as a fantastic solution to some of your most common skin issues, especially acne.

Other Guaranteed Benefits of Intermittent Fasting

Aside from the mentioned health benefits, you will also most likely be encouraged to try IF because of the way it approaches the weight loss process. Here are some of the other benefits of intermittent fasting based on the way it functions:

- **Versatile and flexible** – One thing that makes intermittent fasting stand out from other diet plans and eating patterns is its flexibility. It is so flexible and versatile that you can easily integrate the patterns it uses to any diet.

  You can still fast regardless of what foods you do not eat. For instance, if you do not eat wheat or any wheat-based product, you can still rest assured that intermittent fasting will work for you.

  It is also something that you can do regardless of your lifestyle – whether you are a busy, career-oriented person, a traveler, someone with a strict budget, or one who experiences problems with swallowing or chewing. It is so versatile that you can apply it anytime, anywhere regardless of your lifestyle.

- **Easy to do** – Another fantastic benefit of intermittent fasting is that it is easy and convenient to do. You can do it anytime and anyplace. In case you are unwell due to a certain reason, then you can just stop. You can completely reverse it within just a few minutes.

  The fact that it does not have any set duration also makes it even easier to do and stick to. You are allowed to practice it for as long as you like, maybe as short as 5 or 10 days or longer by doing it for several months.

It does not require you to stick to a very rigid schedule. You are allowed to pick your schedule based on what is convenient for you. For instance, you can choose to fast for several days this week and stop it the next week. You have full control over when you should start this eating pattern and when you should stop, making it all the more convenient.

- **Cheap** – Intermittent fasting also seems to win the hearts of many because this whole approach to weight loss and achieving better health is cheap. While it would be much better if you choose to eat the healthy stuff, like local grass-fed and organic beef, it is not a secret that this organic and natural stuff is quite costly.

  If you try intermittent fasting, then you do not have to spend too much to stay healthy and fit. True, intermittent fasting is not completely free, but you can save a lot of money since you can lessen the number of food you need to buy. You will surely love the fact that IF does not only help you lose weight and stay healthy but also contributes to having huge savings.

- **Does not have extreme limitations in terms of macronutrients** – Intermittent fasting is not like other eating and diet plans that require you to follow dramatic restrictions on certain macronutrients. For instance, some of those who aim to lose weight or improve their health are required to stick strictly to a diet plan low on carbs.

Others, on the other hand, need to stick to a diet, which is low in fat to achieve their weight loss or health goals. These diet programs require you to follow a new manner of eating. In most cases, it requires you to replace the foods you love with unfamiliar and new ones. It may also be inconvenient since you will also have to learn and master new cooking skills.

You do not have to do all that if you decide to go for intermittent fasting. It is because this eating pattern does not have any macronutrient range that you have to target. You do not also need to restrict or forbid certain macronutrients, though, it would still do you good to try eating healthy now and then during your eating window.

Aside from that, intermittent fasting seems to shine because of its simplicity. It is so simple that you will not feel easily discouraged to stick with it. Unlike other diet and weight loss approaches, this eating pattern does not have complex rules and guidelines. This simplicity will promote ease in making it a part of your lifestyle.

Are there Drawbacks (Cons) to Intermittent Fasting?

Intermittent fasting has several benefits to anyone who decides to embrace it. However, just like any other eating pattern or diet plan, which aims is to help you lose weight, it also has its share of drawbacks. Here are just a few of those you have to watch out for.

Low energy

If you are into intermittent fasting, then you will notice the level of your energy dropping every now and then. Remember that food serves as your body's fuel. Because IF requires you to fast, you will not be able to get such fuel from foods especially during your fasting period.

It might cause you to have a significantly low level of energy. Your energy will plummet even during those hours when you are not fasting, especially if the foods you eat during your fed state are not that healthy and energizing. If you notice your energy dropping after you started intermittent fasting, the best way for you to deal with it is to prepare foods that meet your daily nutrient requirements.

Make sure that your body receives all the nutrients it needs. You may also want to take supplements to ensure that your body receives everything it needs to keep working. It is especially important if you are also a vegan or vegetarian.

Intense cravings

Another possible drawback of intermittent fasting is that it might cause you to have intense cravings. You have to observe and monitor these cravings closely as such might indicate something about your body or health. For instance, if you crave red meat, then it could be a sign that you are deficient in iron. If you are craving for citrus fruits, it may also indicate that you need to supply your body with more Vitamin C.

Make sure that you stay fully hydrated once you begin your journey with IF. It is because your hunger or intense cravings may only be caused by thirst instead of hunger. Drink water first before grabbing on whatever it is you want to eat. Be fully hydrated as it can contribute a lot to keeping your appetite under control.

Might cause unwanted or unhealthy food obsession

Another problem with intermittent fasting is that it might cause you to be obsessed with food. The main reason behind this could be your frequent thoughts about when you can eat. You will also feel like you are constantly in a state of alternating extreme restrictions and binging.

If you are not careful, then you will be at risk of having an unhealthy mindset about food. This can result in overeating as well as extreme feelings of shame and guilt every time you overeat.

Might cause grogginess and tiredness

You may experience these negative effects, especially if you are still a beginner in intermittent fasting. Just like what is mentioned earlier, your body's energy will most likely dwindle. Aside from that, fasting might increase your stress level, leading to disruptions in your sleeping patterns.

To avoid feeling extremely tired or groggy because of following the IF protocol, consider doing some activities that might lower your stress level. One of these activities is meditation. If you are working out regularly, it is advisable to schedule it during your fed state. By doing that, you can conserve your energy.

Remember that working out during the time you are fasting is not a good idea as it might only cause your blood sugar to drop too low, causing symptoms like confusion and dizziness. If undealt with, it can make you more prone to injury.

Causes brain fog

Intermittent fasting might also cause brain fog. It is mainly because most of those who are following this habit fast by not eating breakfast. The problem with this, especially if you are still a beginner, is that it might cause fatigue and brain fog. You are even at risk of committing some mistakes because of brain fog. If this happens to you, take it as a sign that you are not consuming healthy foods during your fed state.

In this case, you have to observe what fuels your body in terms of food. Note that while you are allowed to eat the foods you want during your eating hours, you still have to be wise in making your choice. Ensure that your diet still consists mostly of good and healthy foods. Choose healthy foods that can make you feel strong and healthy. Furthermore, they should be able to promote mental clarity.

Results in some menstrual cycle changes

Your menstrual cycle may also have some changes as a result of losing weight immediately due to IF. Women who are doing intermittent fasting and lost a significant amount of weight because of it or were unable to get sufficient calories daily might notice a few changes in their monthly menstrual cycles. Some of them may notice their cycles slowing down or stopping completely.

It is because a sudden loss of weight tends to disrupt your usual hormonal cycles, triggering missed periods. If you notice such changes, especially if your period stopped all of a sudden as a suspected effect of IF, then stop fasting until you have talked to your gynecologist. That way, you can troubleshoot and find out how you can still follow the IF pattern without causing problems on your menstrual cycles.

Other Possible Side Effects

Apart from the drawbacks already mentioned, intermittent fasting might also cause mood swings, headaches, bad breath, and lack of concentration, especially during fasting periods. Most of these side effects are not that serious, though, and tend to go away once you get used to the eating pattern.

In case you have an existing medical condition, it is advisable to talk to your doctor first before adhering to IF. It is even more important for women to consult their doctor, especially if they fall in any of the following:

- Dealt with any form of eating disorder in the past

- Regularly experience low levels of blood sugar

- Diagnosed with diabetes

- Have nutritional deficiencies

- Underweight

- Pregnant and breastfeeding

- Trying to conceive

- Have past or present experiences of missed period or amenorrhea

- Experienced fertility problems

Make sure to get the go-signal of your doctor before you do IF. Note that an excellent safety profile is necessary to make this eating pattern work in your favor. Also, your consultation with your doctor can help you determine if you need to do some modifications for intermittent fasting to provide you with your desired results safely and healthily.

Chapter 3 – Getting Familiar with Different Types of Fasting

One great thing about intermittent fasting is that it provides women with different choices in terms of incorporating this eating pattern into their lifestyle. It is because it comes in different types and patterns. With your multiple options, you can make your choice based on what will work for you. You can also modify it a bit based on the demands of your work and family as well as your available time and resources.

To help you, here are a few of the different types of intermittent fasting that are more likely to work for women:

16/8 Intermittent Fasting Method

One of the most convenient IF methods for women is the 16/8, which involves daily fasting for around fourteen to sixteen hours and an eating window of around eight to ten hours. The 8 to 10-hour eating window is when you can incorporate at least two meals.

Also called the Leangains method, the 16/8 fasting became popular because of its simplicity. It is convenient especially for a lot of busy women since it just involves stopping to eat right after taking dinner and not eating breakfast.

For instance, if your last meal, which is probably dinner, is at 8 pm, then your next meal should be around noon the following day. It should let you fast for a max of 16 hours. For women, though, the most recommended fasting period is 14 to 15 hours as they seem to produce better results when they stick to a bit shorter fasting period.

If you tend to get hungry every morning and are used to eating breakfast, then expect to experience a few challenges when you are still new to it. However, for those who are already used to skipping breakfast, this method is easy for them to follow. During your fasting period, you are allowed to drink coffee and water.

You can also drink other beverages provided they do not have calories. The drinks can be a big help in preventing you from feeling too hungry. Once it is time for you to eat, consider focusing on healthy foods. Note that you can't expect the 16/8 fasting method to work in your favor if you consume junk foods as well as high-calorie foods excessively. You can still eat them but do so in moderation.

Benefits of the 16/8 Intermittent Fasting Method

The 16/8 method is beneficial for a lot of women because aside from being more flexible, it is also not that restrictive. It is so versatile that it is easy to fit it into your lifestyle. It can improve weight loss by restricting your intake of foods to several hours a day.

Aside from that, it lets you fast for a certain period, which can also boost your metabolic rate, a major contributor as far as losing weight is concerned. Furthermore, the 16/8 method also works in improving your ability to control your blood sugar, boosting your longevity, and enhancing your brain function.

How to Do It?

To start this specific intermittent fasting method, choose an 8-hour window that will serve as the period when you should eat. The most convenient method is after dinner, which is usually around 7 to 8 pm since it lets you fast overnight then just easily skip your breakfast the next day. Try to experiment and find out what is the best fasting and eating schedule for you.

To make this method work more favorably for you, consider sticking to whole and nutritious foods and beverages during your eating window. Go for nutrient-rich foods. It would be best to balance every meal with a wide range of whole and nutritious foods, like fruits, whole grains, vegetables, protein-rich foods, and healthy fats.

During your fasting period, try controlling your appetite with healthy drinks, particularly water, calorie-free drinks, and unsweetened coffee and tea. Aside from controlling your appetite, doing so can help you stay hydrated.

Do not binge or overeat junk foods during your eating window, too, as it might only hamper your health and prevent you from getting the results you want from this habit.

5:2 or Fast Diet

You may also want to try the 5:2 or the fast diet. It basically requires you to eat as you normally would five days a week. The remaining two days should have calorie restrictions. It would be best to restrict your intake of calories in the two days left to just around 500 to 600.

As a guide, your calorie restriction should be 25% of the usual amount your body takes in, which is often around 500 to 600 calories. This method also often requires you to separate the two fasting days. You can do so by having a day in between each fasting day.

Benefits of the 5:2 or Fast Diet

One great thing about the 5:2 or the fast diet is that it does not have huge limitations in terms of food. This means that you can't consider any food as off-limits. It is the reason why it appeals to a lot of people, especially women, who are aiming to improve their general health and well-being as well as slim down. Apart from weight loss, the 5:2 or fast diet is also known for preventing and managing diabetes as well as improving the health of your heart. It is also good for your brain and cognitive health.

How to Do It?

To start with the 5:2 or fast diet, you can pick your fasting days. The good thing about this IF method is that it gives you the freedom to pick the two days when you should fast depending on your schedule. Experiment with timing so you can identify the specific schedule that will work favorably for both your body and brain.

As for the 5 days when you should eat, make sure to eat normally. It does not necessarily mean overeating, though. You just have to eat based on what your body needs. Do not overeat, especially overly processed, sugary, and high-calorie foods as doing so may only prevent you from losing weight.

As for fasting, keep in mind that you only have limited calories to take in. Spread out your allowed calorie intake over the two fasting days. You can eat high-volume foods to achieve that. For instance, if you need to take in 500 calories during your fasting day, you can divide it by eating 200 calories each during breakfast and dinner then 100 calories at lunch.

Take note, though, that if you are still new to this form of fasting, you may experience a few negative side effects, like nausea, mood swings, weakness, headaches, fatigue, sleepiness, and irritability. You do not have to worry too much as these side effects are just minor.

You can also expect these negative side effects to go away once you get used to this IF method. However, if you still find these issues overwhelming, then you can rest assured that you can handle them through simple ways, like drinking more water, taking a bath or shower, stretching, taking a nap, staying busy, and meditating.

Eat-Stop-Eat

Also referred to as the 24-hour IF protocol, the eat-stop-eat involves fasting for the full 24 hours one or two times every week. For women, a max of twice per week eat-stop-eat fasting is highly recommended. If you are still new, then you may want to start with fasting periods of just 14 to 16 hours then slowly build it up.

You are allowed to eat normally during the days of the week when you are not fasting. However, during your fasting days, you need to stay away from solid foods and drinks containing any calories. One thing to note about eat-stop-eat is that it is not your usual diet for weight loss. It involves reevaluating your present knowledge about meal frequency and timing and its connection to your health.

Benefits of Eat-Stop-Eat

One amazing benefit of this specific approach to intermittent fasting is that it does not involve starving yourself every day. It is because you are allowed to eat anything for 5 or 6 days weekly. It, therefore, comes with flexible timing, which still lets you enjoy the foods you love.

You can still have breakfast with the people you love, enjoy a dinner date with your partner, or attend parties. Aside from that, it may also promote weight loss since it involves prolonged fasting periods.

How to Do It?

Eat-stop-eat involves a straightforward approach. To implement it, you just have to pick one to two days every week, preferably non-consecutive, when you should fast or abstain from eating for 24 hours straight.

Allow yourself to enjoy the foods you love during the remaining non-fasting days. However, it is still advisable to make wise and sensible food choices. Do not take in more than what your body needs. You also have to remember the importance of proper hydration during fasting days.

This means you have to drink enough water during each scheduled 24-hour fasting period. You can also hydrate by drinking calorie-free beverages, like artificially sweetened or unsweetened tea or coffee.

Crescendo Fasting

The crescendo fasting method also works well for women who want to try intermittent fasting. It is different from the usual IF protocols that require you to fast for around 12 to 20 hours daily. In crescendo fasting, you will need to cut down your fasting period to just 12 to 16 hours.

You have to do the fasting for around 2-3 times weekly. Make sure that the fasting days are not consecutive. The primary intention of crescendo fasting is to increase the level of fasting your body can take slowly.

Benefits of Crescendo Fasting

Crescendo fasting is beneficial because it involves a gentler approach that works suitably for a woman's body. This technique works hand in hand with your hormones in a gentle manner in order to retain a healthy balance. With that, expect it to help in keeping your energy and metabolism up.

It also contributes to losing body fat. This method requires you to fast in less frequent and shorter bursts, so it can lower your calorie intake without causing your body to be in a stressful state caused by starvation. This specific practice can initiate weight loss.

How to Do It?

To take full advantage of crescendo fasting, it is advisable to do the fasting on alternate days, preferably two to three non-consecutive days every week. For instance, if you plan to set aside 3 days for fasting, then you can schedule it on Mondays, Wednesdays, and Saturdays. Each fasting period should take around 12 to 16 hours.

It helps to take branched-chain amino acids (BCAAs) supplement during your fasting days. This supplement plays several important functions like satisfying your hunger, supporting protein synthesis, reducing muscle damage, speeding up the healing process, and offering help when it comes to building new muscle tissues. It is also advisable to do light exercises, instead of intense and rigorous ones when you are fasting.

Another important component of this intermittent fasting approach is proper hydration. This means that whether you are on your fasting or eating days, you have to supply your body with enough water. It is highly recommended to consume a minimum of 64 ounces of water every day but you are also allowed to have coffee and tea every now and then. If possible, choose those beverages without artificial sweeteners or additional sugars, too.

The Warrior Diet

The Warrior diet refers to an eating pattern or intermittent fasting method, which involves cycling prolonged periods of small food consumption with short periods of overeating. It is an approach, which many consider as effective when it comes to weight loss as well as improving mental clarity and energy levels.

The food choices in this eating pattern are somewhat the same as those you can eat in the Paleo diet. This means that it mostly consists of unprocessed and whole foods.

Benefits of the Warrior Diet

Although the whole premise of the Warrior diet is more extreme compared to the other IF methods, you will still be pleased to know that it carries several incredible benefits – one of which is weight loss. One reason behind this is that you can significantly lower your calorie intake when you are following this approach.

Another possible advantage of the Warrior diet is improved brain health. It is mainly because this fasting method regulates inflammatory pathways that have a great impact on the way your brain functions.

Moreover, this IF approach is also known for reducing inflammation that might cause several diseases, like diabetes and heart disease. You will also feel more in control of your blood sugar level if you stick to the Warrior diet for quite a long time.

How to Do It?

For the Warrior diet to work to your advantage, timing is essential. It should be based on the premise that you have to fast for a long period and set a shorter eating window to improve your health, body composition, and fitness.

The fasting period should take 20 hours. During this period, you should take in only minimal calories. You can sustain yourself during this period with tiny portions of raw produce, hard-boiled eggs, and dairy. You are also allowed to drink beverages with zero-calorie content. You can also drink coffee even during your fasting hours.

Once your feeding window comes, you are allowed to eat anything. Just make sure to do eat only within the 4-hour eating window. To ensure that you can conveniently practice this eating pattern, consider basing your feeding window on a certain timeframe that is favorable for you.

Most of those who follow this approach swear to the effectiveness of scheduling the 4-hour feast or eating window during the evening, though. Find out if this schedule works for you. If it does, then you can stick to it.

Modified Alternate-Day Fasting

This form of IF involves a fasting schedule of every other day. You are then allowed to eat normally during non-fasting days. This approach also lets you consume around 20 to 25 percent of the calories you consume usually around 500 calories during the days when you are fasting.

Benefits of the Modified Alternate-Day Fasting

Modified alternate-day fasting is a good IF approach for several women because of its weight loss benefits. This means that it can assist you during your journey towards losing weight. Some of those who follow this approach also say that it can help lessen waist circumference as well as your blood pressure, triglycerides, and bad cholesterol. You will also find the modified alternate-day fasting method effective in preventing or managing Type 2 diabetes.

How to Do It?

As mentioned earlier, the main idea behind modified alternate-day fasting is to set aside one day of fasting then eating whatever you want the next day. You have to alternate fasting and eating days to make it work in your favor. With this approach, you only have to limit the foods you want to eat half of the time.

During your scheduled fasting days, drinking as many beverages without calories as you want is allowed. Some examples of these drinks are water, tea, and unsweetened coffee. Also, remember that the modified alternate-day fasting technique lets you consume around 500 calories during your fasting days. This should make up around 20 to 25 percent of your energy needs.

There are indeed several approaches and techniques that you can apply if you want to do intermittent fasting. However, no matter which one you choose, it is still advisable to be wise during your eating windows or non-fasting days or hours. Yes, you are allowed to eat anything during that period, but it would still be best to choose your foods wisely based on their health benefits.

Keep in mind that if you consume huge amounts of calorie-dense and unhealthy foods once your eating window comes, then it would be harder for you to get the health benefits and weight loss you are hoping for.

Also, remember how important it is to follow an IF technique that you can manage and tolerate. It should be something that you can sustain for quite a long time. Make sure that your chosen approach does not have negative consequences on your health, too.

Chapter 4 – Foods to Eat and Avoid When you are on IF

Now that you know the different types of intermittent fasting that you can implement, it is time to pick the one that is most favorable for you. Figure out which one fits your requirements the most as well as your current health, weight, and lifestyle. Once you have made your choice on an IF approach or method to follow, it is advisable to learn a thing or two about making wise and healthy food choices.

Remember that it would be impossible for you to generate the specific results you want from intermittent fasting if you constantly fill your body with unhealthy stuff. Yes, IF allows you to lose weight while still enjoying the foods you love during your eating window. However, that does not necessarily mean that you should go for unhealthy stuff entirely.

To help make the most out of each eating window, it is crucial to get an idea about the foods you are allowed to eat as well as those you need to stay away from. This specific chapter will cover such information, so you will be a more informed practitioner of intermittent fasting.

Foods to Eat When Following Intermittent Fasting

As mentioned earlier, intermittent fasting is an eating pattern that does not have extreme restrictions on the foods you can eat during your eating window.

However, you can do yourself a great favor if you still try to be wise in making food choices. As much as possible, pick only the healthy stuff. Here are just some of the foods you can eat if you are interested to follow intermittent fasting and maximize its positive effects:

Foods Rich in Lean Protein

Anyone who wants to maximize the effects of intermittent fasting should incorporate various sources of lean protein into their diet plans. This means that during their eating window, they should eat foods rich in lean protein, like lean beef, seafood, and chicken. Eggs are also excellent sources of lean and healthy protein.

The great thing about eggs is that you can easily and quickly prepare them. You can also get lean protein from chicken breast, lentils, peas, beans, tempeh, plain Greek yogurt, and tofu.

You need to supply your body with enough lean protein as it allows you to feel full longer, which helps you survive fasting periods. Aside from that, lean protein contributes to muscle-building, which also plays a major role in boosting your metabolism.

Fruits and Berries

It is also advisable to include fruits and berries in your diet. Do not overload on fruit, though, as they also have plenty of natural sugar, which might interfere with the level of your insulin. The key here is to make wise choices regarding the fruits you can incorporate into your diet.

As much as possible, focus more on eating berries because they have high antioxidant and nutritional content. You can even add berries together with nuts into your salad to let your body receive a wide range of nutrients in just one serving. To help you craft delicious meal plans, here are some fruits and berries that you can safely eat while on IF:

- **Raspberries** – Among the healthiest fruits that you can eat while following intermittent fasting are raspberries. One advantage of raspberries is that these fruits are rich in fiber. Each cup of it can even supply you with up to 8 grams of fiber. It is a delicious fruit with high fiber content, which can help you stay regular when trying to stick to a shortened feeding or eating window.

- **Blueberries** – Blueberries are also great additions to your diet as they are rich in antioxidants that promote youthfulness and longevity. The fact that these fruits are rich in antioxidants helps in getting rid of free radicals from your body, thereby preventing widespread cell damage. They are also among the healthiest snacks you can grab during your eating window.

- **Papaya** – Another fruit that is safe to eat when trying to adhere to the intermittent fasting approach is papaya. It is a great fruit to eat, especially if you are still a beginner in IF and you often feel hunger and its effects at the remaining hours of your long fasting period.

Note that such hunger might cause you to overeat, leading to bloating and lethargy afterward. You can eat papaya to relieve the discomfort brought on by that scenario. It is because of the unique enzyme in papaya called papain, which acts on protein by breaking it down.

A wise tip is to include chunks of papaya, a tropical fruit, into a protein-dense meal. It can benefit you in the sense that it will ease digestion, promoting ease in managing the bloat.

- **Avocado** – You can also greatly benefit from eating avocado while on IF. You do not have to worry about it being rich in calories because it also has monounsaturated fat, which is known for being extremely satiating.

  With that, you have an assurance that it can help you stay full for longer. You can include half of this fruit into your lunch to experience its satiating effects. Because it makes you feel full, you can manage your fasting hours even better.

Other healthy fruits that you can eat when following IF are apricots, cherries, apples, blackberries, oranges, pears, peaches, plums, and watermelon.

Leafy and Cruciferous Vegetables

Vegetables also play a vital role in your intermittent fasting regimen. You have to include leafy greens in your diet as it has plenty of health benefits, including lowering your risk of dealing with cognitive decline, Type 2 diabetes, heart disease, and cancer.

Cruciferous vegetables, like Brussels sprouts, cauliflower, and broccoli, can also greatly benefit intermittent fasting practitioners because of their high fiber content. By eating foods rich in fiber, you can improve your digestion and ensure that you become full faster and longer.

The fullness you can get from it is a good thing, especially if you need to fast for long hours. Aside from that, the high fiber content present in cruciferous vegetables can also help prevent constipation. Other veggies that you have to include in your diet are kale, chard, arugula, collard greens, cabbage, and spinach.

Seafood

You should also try to include a serving of seafood into your diet. Seafood is rich in nutrients, particularly Omega-3 fatty acids that can make you less prone to suffering from depression, dementia, and heart disease. You should eat fish regularly because aside from supplying your body with protein and healthy fats, it is also rich in Vitamin D.

The fact that seafood, particularly fish, is rich in nutrients can also benefit you, especially if you want your foods to be truly nutritious since you only have a limited eating window. Seafood, including fish, shrimp, trout, and salmon are also nutrient-dense brain foods. They can even help boost your cognitive function.

Whole Grains

You also have a higher chance of enjoying favorable results from intermittent fasting if you consume whole grains during your eating window. Whole grains have high protein and fiber content, which means that even if you eat just a little of it, you will experience fullness.

Apart from that, whole grains can improve your metabolism, which can help you in your attempt to lose weight. Some of those you ought to try are whole grain bread and rice, sorghum, millet, spelt, bulgur, amaranth, and farro.

White Potatoes

White potatoes are also among the foods you can eat. The good thing about potatoes is that your body can easily digest them with the least effort. If you work out regularly, then you can pair white potatoes with a source of protein. Such a combination can make a great post-workout snack, which can refuel your tired muscles.

White potatoes are also great additions to the IF diet because once they cool down, they can create a resistant starch, which can help in fueling the good bacteria found in your gut. You can also expect white potatoes to support weight loss. However, keep in mind that potato chips and French fries are not among those that can provide such a benefit.

Beans and Legumes

You should also consider making beans and legumes a part of your IF lifestyle and diet if you want to make the most out of it. The good thing about beans and legumes, like black beans, peas, and chickpeas, is that they can elevate your energy. These foods are also great sources of energy.

Being categorized as low-calorie carbs, they are perfect if you want to supply your body with just enough carbs. Aside from that, beans and legumes can reduce body weight without restricting your calorie intake too much.

Nuts

Eating nuts while on IF can also greatly benefit your body. Among those nutritious nuts, you can make a part of your IF diet are hazelnuts, walnuts, cashews, and almonds. You can eat them as healthy snacks. While it is true that nuts have high-calorie content, they are still healthy snacks because they contain good fats. Moreover, nuts are rich in antioxidants.

What can You Drink?

Apart from foods, you also have to get an idea about the safest beverages you can drink when trying to follow intermittent fasting. Ensure that you stick to the following beverages to ensure that you get your desired results from IF:

- **Water** – Note that a vital aspect when trying to commit to a healthy eating pattern when doing IF is proper hydration. Keep in mind that the eating pattern will let you go on with your daily activities even without fuel. It is because you might need to fast for around 12 to 24 hours.

In that case, the source of energy preferred by your body is glycogen, the stored sugar in your liver. Upon burning such stored energy, it is also possible for a huge volume of electrolytes and fluid to diminish, leading to dehydration.

With that in mind, ensure that you drink around 8 cups or more of water daily. It is a big help in preventing dehydration. By ensuring that you are well-hydrated, you can also expect better cognition, joint and muscle support, and blood flow, which has a positive impact on your IF regimen.

- **Coffee** – Being on IF also allows you to enjoy a cup or two of your favorite coffee. The good news is that just like water, you can drink it even outside of your scheduled feeding window. It is because when it comes in its natural form, coffee is devoid of calories.

  However, you have to be extra careful because creamers, syrups, and candied flavorings are not allowed during your fasting period. Keep that restriction in mind so you will not end up making such a mistake when it is still time for you to fast.

- **Tea** – Tea is also naturally free of calories, so it is okay for you to drink it during your fasting period. Just make sure that you choose brewed tea derived from tea leaves, flakes, or bags. Stay away from bottled iced tea as much as possible as it tends to have heavy doses of sugar and other sweeteners. Just like what is recommended on coffee, you should also reserve caloric add-ons, such as cream, milk, or honey during your eating window.

- **Bone or vegetable broth** – You can also drink this one in case your fasting period lasts for at least 24 hours. Be extra careful with bouillon cubes and canned broths, though, as they contain plenty of preservatives and artificial flavors that might only ruin the positive results of your fast. Choose a homemade broth, instead, one that comes from a reliable and trusted source.

- **Almond milk** – One advantage of almond milk is that it tends to have low calorie and carb content. One cup of it has only around 39 calories, so it is a great drink when fasting.

  You can consume up to 100 ml of this drink when fasting, so you will feel fuller and more satisfied. It can also provide your body with essential minerals as well as Vitamin E. Just make sure to stay away from almond milk with added sugar.

What Foods and Drinks to Avoid?

Now that you have an idea of the specific foods and drinks you are allowed to eat and drink when trying to stick to an IF method, it is time to get to know what you should avoid. By knowing exactly what you should stay away from, you can prevent yourself from consuming anything that may just ruin the effects of intermittent fasting on you. Here are those you should avoid:

- Processed foods and meat

- Alcoholic beverages

- Sugar-sweetened drinks

- Refined grains

- Candy bars, sweets, and other sugary foods

- Foods rich in trans fat

- Fast food

Some Tips to Keep in Mind

When creating your meal plans that adhere to the intermittent fasting lifestyle, make sure to keep in mind the foods and drinks you can consume and should avoid. You can also craft better diet plans while keeping in mind the principles of IF with these tips:

- **Get carbs from healthy sources** – These include fruits, beans, grains, and veggies that are rich in fiber. By doing that, you can slow down sugar absorption in your bloodstream.

- **Stick to a diverse diet containing nutrient-dense foods** – These include high-fiber carbs, such as fruits, veggies, and whole grains, as well as healthy fats and lean proteins. Make sure that your meals consist of the three important macronutrients.

By doing that, you have an assurance that you will feel energized and satisfied during your fasting period. A guide for getting macronutrient balance is 45% carbs, 25 % healthy fats, and 30% protein.

- **Divide your eating window into multiple meals and snacks** – A wise advice is to plan your eating window in a way that you can eat two large meals, as well as two or three small snacks. Such is enough to supply your body with enough nutrients and energy, preventing you from feeling unsatisfied and famished.

- **Try limiting your sources of protein to fish or poultry** – You can cook it in fat or consume the poultry skin. Also, try restricting your intake of protein to the thickness and size of your palm.

- **Stay hydrated** – Remember that it is common for anyone to mistake thirst with hunger. You can prevent misinterpreting your thirst by ensuring that you remain well-hydrated all the time.

  Start your day with a glass of water. Drink it upon waking up. Make sure that you also drink water every now and then during your fasting period. What's great about drinking enough water is that it also works in suppressing your appetite.

- **Add flavor to beverages without calories** – Doing so can further encourage you to continue and finish the fasting period. Make it a point to drink naturally flavored water, unsweetened iced or hot tea, black coffee, or seltzer. In case you have a hard time taking in black coffee, you may want to add unsweetened cocoa, Stevia, or cinnamon to it.

With proper planning and careful research, you can surely create a diet plan, which adheres to the guidelines set by your chosen IF method. By including the right foods and removing unwanted ones from your diet plan, you can achieve whatever result you are hoping to get from IF, including weight loss.

Chapter 5 – Who can Benefit from Intermittent Fasting?

Before trying out intermittent fasting, you have to find out whether it will work for you first. You have to determine if this eating pattern is appropriate for you first based on your present weight, lifestyle, body type, and health condition.

Note that even if it has plenty of benefits when done properly, like regulating your blood glucose, managing your body weight, gaining or maintaining lean muscle mass, and controlling blood lipids, it is not suitable for everyone. If you are still unsure, you may want to consult your doctor first.

Seek his advice and find out if your health will not get drastically affected by your decision to try intermittent fasting. In most cases, though, intermittent fasting seems to produce favorable and successful results for those who have the following or belong to any of the following:

- Have a history of monitoring food and calorie intake

- Has enough experience in terms of working out

- Single or does not have children

- Have a supportive partner – someone who supports your decision to try IF

- Have a job that lets you have low-performance periods while adapting to a new eating pattern or plan

- Obtained a go-signal from their doctor to try IF

Intermittent fasting can also greatly benefit those who intend to lose weight. In fact, weight loss is one factor that encouraged most practitioners of this eating pattern to give it a try.

However, take note that while there are those who can greatly benefit from intermittent fasting, some should also avoid it as much as possible. It does not seem to work well for those who are underweight or dealt with eating disorders in the past. You can still try it, though, but you have to get the go-signal of a health professional first.

It is not also highly recommended for those who are:

- Pregnant

- Suffering from chronic stress

- Have sleeping disorders

- Still new in terms of dieting and exercising

If you are still a beginner when it comes to dieting and working out, you may think that intermittent fasting is the best solution for you if your goal is to lose weight. However, you have to be wise enough to address all possible nutritional deficiencies first before experimenting with your fast. Start with a solid nutritional platform if you are truly serious about doing intermittent fasting.

Also, remember that hunger is one of the major side effects of IF. It might also cause you to feel weak or lower the performance of your brain. Fortunately, these effects are usually only temporary. You will most likely experience them only while your body is still adapting to your new habits and eating patterns.

However, if you are suffering from a medical condition, seeking the advice of your doctor first is a must. Your doctor's opinion is even more important if you have diabetes, issues with regulating blood sugar, and low blood pressure.

Should You Give It a Try?

One great thing about intermittent fasting is that it boasts of an outstanding safety profile. Fasting for a while will not cause you any harm provided you are well-nourished and healthy overall. If you are still trying to figure out if you can greatly benefit from it, then find out if you meet the following criteria:

- Your relationship with food is healthy.

- You are capable of controlling your eating habits after breaking the fast.

- Your mental sharpness and productivity are not affected by fasting.

- You have good health overall.

- You have low or manageable stress levels.

The best way to determine if intermittent fasting is good for you is to try it for a while. If you still feel great even when you are fasting, and you discover that this approach is a more sustainable eating solution for you, then you can view it as a truly powerful tool for your weight loss journey.

You can even use it to improve your health. Also, remember that there are certain factors that you have to focus on to maximize its benefits including your workouts, sleeping patterns, and healthy eating habits.

What Body Type can Benefit More from Intermittent Fasting?

As mentioned earlier, you can't expect intermittent fasting to work for everyone. The principles, patterns, and guidelines behind it do not suit all body types, too. It should be noted that there are three basic body types. There is the mesomorph, which is characterized by a solid and strong build.

Those who have this body type are usually not underweight nor overweight. They seem to have rectangular body shapes and come with upright postures. Mesomorphs also have muscular legs and arms, muscular shoulders and chest, and even weight distribution.

Since mesomorphs do not often experience trouble eating whatever they want because they tend to lose weight easily, they may have an easier time crafting the perfect diet plan for them. However, they also tend to gain weight readily. In that case, intermittent fasting will surely work for them as this allows them to eat whatever they want during the eating window without worrying about their weight suddenly increasing.

Another body type that you have to be aware of is the endomorph. The endomorph body type is often characterized by less muscles and body fats. This is the reason why those with this body type usually look soft and round. They also tend to put on pounds quickly and easily.

However, take note that being an endomorph does not necessarily mean you are already overweight. It is just that this body type tends to gain more weight easily than the others. It is also quick and easy for endomorphs to increase their strength and build muscles.

If you have this body type, then a wise tip when it comes to dieting is to try reducing your carb intake. It is also advisable to increase your intake of water and other healthy beverages for proper hydration. It is also important to note that endomorphs respond better to intermittent fasting compared to the other body types.

With that in mind, it is no longer surprising to see IF being the go-to solution for endomorphs who are trying to lose weight or maintain a fit body. Intermittent fasting also seems to work more effectively for endomorphs based on their metabolic rate.

The last body type is the ectomorph. You can see ectomorphs having a thinner body and lower weight and longer limbs. Compared to endomorphs, ectomorphs have a more accelerated metabolism. It is also not easy for them to gain muscles, though it is necessary for them to perform certain exercises to improve their strength.

If you are an ectomorph, then know that your metabolism is different from endomorphs. In this case, intermittent fasting is not a good fit for your body type. It is the reason why it is not highly recommended for them. As far as body type is concerned, IF seems to work more suitably for endomorphs.

Chapter 6 – Intermittent Fasting and Pregnancy: Is IF Safe for Pregnant Women?

One of the most common concerns of women who are currently doing IF or are still planning to make the eating pattern a part of their lifestyle is its possible effects in case they get pregnant. You may start asking yourself, "what if I get pregnant?". Can I still fast? Is intermittent fasting safe for me when I am already pregnant or trying to get pregnant?

Remember that if you get pregnant, then your body can grow and change. You will notice these changes happening faster, especially as you move closer to the date of your delivery. Some changes in your body during pregnancy can be a bit disconcerting.

However, if you are greatly concerned that the weight you have put on is already too much, then it is necessary to find out how you can manage it the healthy way. You may start wondering if it is still okay for you to do intermittent fasting to manage your weight or deal with any health concern.

If you are someone who practices intermittent fasting, then you would surely want to know if this practice is something you can continue during the months of your pregnancy. To eliminate your confusion, the first thing you have to do is to contact your doctor first. Ask him about how safe IF is for your pregnancy before you start changing your eating habits.

Is IF Recommended During Pregnancy?

Generally, intermittent fasting is not recommended for pregnant women. However, take note that no informed recommendations are out yet regarding its negative or positive effects on pregnancy. Most of the studies that link fasting and pregnancy usually revolve around Ramadan, which is a Muslim holiday that lasts for around 30 days. This is the time when Muslims fast the entire day.

Note that technically, those who are breastfeeding and pregnant are exempted from fasting. However, there are still those who fast even if they are pregnant. Most of those who still fast during pregnancy experienced huge changes in the level of their triglyceride, insulin, and glucose.

The birth weight of babies delivered by those who fasted, though, is usually comparable to the birth weight of babies of moms who did not fast. Despite that, there are still researchers who claim that fasting when pregnant might have health consequences in the future.

If you are thinking of fasting to manage your weight during pregnancy, you can take note of the studies and research made on IF. Also, do not forget that pregnancy is the time for you to prioritize things, like helping your baby develop and gain weight, supplying enough nutrition to your baby for proper body and brain development, and forming maternal fat stores in case you intend to breastfeed.

With that in mind, you should avoid making dramatic changes in your eating habits as it might lead to nutritional deficiencies as well as other health issues. There is also a possibility for fasting to change the level of your hormones.

While it is not completely banned from the diet plans of pregnant women because those who are particularly healthy seem to handle this eating pattern well, it is still important to give it a go only after you have received the clearance or go-signal from your doctor. Also, be knowledgeable about your health.

If you are diabetic even before you got pregnant or you are diagnosed with gestational diabetes, a type of diabetes that develops only during pregnancy, then intermittent fasting is not recommended for you. It is because fasting has a negative effect on the level of your blood sugar.

If you fast during the day, then there is a great possibility for the level of your blood sugar to drop significantly. It might also lead to dehydration. If you break your fast during the evening, then you are prone to having extremely high blood sugar levels, especially if you eat a lot at dawn and dusk. With that in mind, you should try to avoid fasting if you are pregnant who also has diabetes.

What are the Usual Risks or Safety Concerns?

If you received your doctor's go-signal, then maybe you can start doing IF, although it is best not to do this practice as intensely as you did before. Also, be extra observant of your body. It is because while there are still no clear answers as to the long-term implications of IF to pregnant women, it has been discovered among women who fast for Ramadan that this habit tends to affect fetal breathing.

It is mainly because fasting can significantly lower your glucose level, which might cause you to spend a much longer time to sense or detect fetal movements, like breathing. Note that infrequent fetal movements are usually warning signs that something is happening inside. This is especially true if your delivery date is already close.

If you are still fasting during pregnancy, then make sure to keep track of your baby's movements. Count his movements. He should be able to make around ten movements in a span of one to two hours. In most cases, you can feel such movements in just thirty minutes.

Another risk you have to take note of is that you may have a hard time supplying your body with the nutrients you need during your feeding window. It is mainly because the time you will eat is restricted to certain days or windows. It is even harder since your baby tends to pull even your nutrition stores.

Aside from that, keep in mind that pregnant women are already prone to experiencing problems such as iron deficiency anemia. The main problem here is that if your baby is unable to get an adequate supply of iron, especially during your third trimester, then there is a great possibility for him to develop anemia.

Fortunately, you can prevent that from happening by ensuring that you only eat the healthiest and most nutritious foods during your eating windows. Try not to be so drastic about your intermittent fasting approach, too. For instance, you should be lenient on your fasting periods by keeping it shorter than usual.

Some Warning Signs You Have to Watch Out For

One of the most important things you have to do when doing IF during your pregnancy is to observe your body. Keep track of your health and what you are feeling, especially during your fasting hours. By monitoring everything that you feel, you can immediately take action, especially if you notice something that might be harmful to you and your baby.

Make sure that you call your midwife or doctor and ask for advice immediately if you experience any of the following when you are fasting:

- **You experience some weight issues** – It could be that you do not put on the recommended weight gain or you are losing too much weight. These issues may harm the development of your baby.

  It would be best for you to weigh yourself regularly. Do not wait for your prenatal appointments to get your weight. By weighing regularly at home, you will know if you have problems with your weight caused by IF that might negatively affect your baby.

- **You have signs of dehydration** – Among the signs of dehydration you have to watch out for are extreme thirst, less frequent urination, and dark-colored urine. It is important to make sure that you are properly hydrated during the entire duration of your pregnancy. It is because dehydration might cause you to suffer from urinary tract infections and other complications that pregnant women are prone to developing.

- **You feel faint or dizzy** – This might also be accompanied by confusion, extreme tiredness, and weakness even if you have enough sleep and rest. If you experience any of the mentioned issues, it is advisable to break your fast right away. You can do so by consuming a sugary beverage or a snack. You should also contact your doctor right away if what you are feeling is somewhat intense.

If you are pregnant and serious about following the IF lifestyle, it is necessary to observe your body well. Listen to your body and determine if you feel anything that is quite alarming. If possible, do not fast for an extremely long time as it might have an impact on your baby's development.

It would be best to avoid implementing IF techniques with fasting periods that last for at least 24 hours. Go for shorter ones. Also, make it a point to decide on whether you should do IF or not based on your present health condition, your baby's development, and how safe you feel.

Chapter 7 – How Pregnant Women can Maximize the Effects of IF?

While not completely recommended, those who seriously want to consider implementing intermittent fasting during their pregnancy would love to know that it shows no or just little effect on newborn babies. However, remember that you, as the one who fasts while pregnant, may have to deal with certain side effects, like lack of energy and dehydration.

To cope with IF well during your pregnancy, you have to keep in mind the following facts related to fasting:

- It does not make you more prone to delivering the baby prematurely.

- It does not cause lower than the usual birth weight.

- It might lead to a lower level of energy. This usually happens during your fasting period since you will most likely not consume as much water and food as your body needs.

- Fasting once you reach your second trimester may lead to a lower risk of gestational diabetes. You may also avoid gaining too much weight by implementing it.

Also, keep in mind that if your weight is healthy during the start of your pregnancy and you have already practiced a healthy lifestyle and diet in the past, then you will have an easier time coping with fasting. Yes, your baby requires certain nutrients but if you already have enough energy stores, then each fasting period will have less to zero impact on your baby.

Another important thing you have to constantly remind yourself of is that the way your body responds to intermittent fasting depends on several factors – among which are your overall health and fitness before you got pregnant, your present pregnancy stage, and the specific length of time you fast. The length can range from 11 to 18 hours.

As much as possible, keep the fasting period shorter to avoid drastic effects on your body and energy level. You can also better cope with the fasting period with the help of these tips:

- **Talk to a healthcare provider or doctor first** – This tip is always worth reiterating just to ensure that you and your baby will stay safe. Have your health checked by a health professional first. Remember that being pregnant is a demanding period for your body.

  Before you start implementing IF, talk to your doctor first. Try to work out with him so you can determine your specific dietary requirements. If possible, visit your doctor often once you begin your IF while pregnant journey, so your condition and that of your baby will be regularly checked up.

  Talking to your doctor is even more important if you are diagnosed with diabetes and still plan to fast. That way, you and your doctor can carefully plan the foods and drinks that you can safely consume.

- **Use a food diary** – Make sure that you also have a food diary around. List down anything that you eat and drink during your eating windows. It will give you an idea of what you put inside your body. By knowing the foods and drinks you regularly take in, you can determine whether you still need to make adjustments on your diet.

- **Stay hydrated** – Remember the importance of staying hydrated when you are fasting. It is especially important during warm weather. Ensure that you get at least 8 glasses of water daily and hydrate even further by eating foods with plenty of water during your eating window. Some great options are soups and stews.

- **Increase your intake of foods rich in fiber** – When breaking your fast or during your eating window, make sure that you eat foods rich in fiber. Some examples are fruits, beans, whole grains, and vegetables. It is because the changes you have made to your eating patterns and habits as well as the lack of fluid might lead to constipation. You can avoid that by adding more fiber to your diet.

- **Eat small meals often** – Do this during your eating window. Have small yet frequent meals during your non-fasting periods to prevent indigestion, which usually happens if you fasting. Avoid eating foods with high sodium (salt) or fat content, though, as those might also cause problems with digestion when you are practicing IF.

- **Do not overwork yourself** – Remember that being pregnant requires you to go easy on doing stuff that requires you to exert a lot of effort. It means to try to reduce housework or lessen those tasks that often tire you out. You should also avoid carrying heavy stuff or walking long distances. Try doing only light tasks, especially during your fasting hours since your energy is most likely not that high in that period.

- **Begin your eating window with light meals** – Among your choices are soups. You can also eat foods with natural sugar, like milk-based drinks and fruits. By starting your eating window with light foods and drinks, instead of gobbling a huge meal right away, you can slowly break the fast, prevent indigestion, and get a good supply of your needed energy.

- **Eat a balanced meal** – You can also better cope with intermittent fasting while pregnant if you make sure that your meals are all healthy and well-balanced. A wise tip is to prepare your meals in a way that they consist of a healthy balance of fruits, veggies, starchy foods, and dairy products.

Your meals should also consist of protein-based foods, like fish, beans, eggs, and well-cooked lean meat. This can provide your body with nutrients that your baby can use for his proper growth and development.

- **Go for complex carbs** – Your meals should also consist of foods with complex carbs. Some examples of these foods are whole grains and seeds. You also need to consume more fiber, like the one you get from dried fruits and pulses.

  By supplying your body with enough complex carbs and fiber, you will have the energy to keep going since they have the ability to release energy gradually. It is also advisable to go for healthier alternatives to refined and high-fat foods. Some great examples are chickpeas and potatoes.

- **Stay away from sugary foods** – Make sure that you do not eat excessive amounts of foods rich in sugar. It is because these food choices can quickly elevate then drop down the level of your blood sugar. If unmanaged, it might lead to dizziness that might cause you to faint.

With the help of these tips, you can better manage your eating patterns while following intermittent fasting during your pregnancy. Another helpful tip is to never feel guilty just in case you choose to stop IF, especially if you have been doing it way before you got pregnant.

Get rid of the guilt even if fasting is part of your religion during holidays. Note that most religious faiths allow nursing and expectant moms to not fast for a while. After all, your health and that of your baby should be on top of your priorities. Your decision should always be based on what you and your doctor think and feel like the safest route for you.

What Can You Do Instead of IF?

If your doctor advises you against intermittent fasting while pregnant or you feel like you can't do it because of safety concerns, then you can rest assured that there are things you can do to stay healthy and fit during your entire pregnancy. One thing you should constantly remind yourself of when planning to maintain a steady and healthy weight gain is to set a target calorie intake of 300 extra calories daily.

Note that you only need a bit of extra, and you can already get that from one-half of a sandwich and one glass of milk. This means that being pregnant does not necessarily mean that you have to eat for two. You just have to put in additional calories for you and your baby's health and development.

Exercise should also form part of the picture. While pregnancy might make you feel sluggish, especially during the first three months, it is still advisable to move your body regularly. It does not have to be intense. You can go for mild exercises or movements.

By exercising regularly, you can prevent gestational diabetes, which tends to develop on some pregnant women. It is also a big help in shortening the number of hours you spent on labor and lowering your risk of having a cesarean delivery.

If you are already fond of working out before you got pregnant, then that's great news. You may ask your obstetrician or doctor if there are things that you have to modify or change on your routines now. If you are still a beginner in working out, then you can stick to around thirty minutes of moderate physical activities daily. Some examples are swimming, cycling on your stationary bike, and walking.

You may also want to tweak your meal plans a bit, especially the ones you are following before when you were still so committed to following the IF protocol. Note that being pregnant does not necessarily mean you have to eat every waking hour. Note that in accordance with your health and pregnancy, which is based on whether you are gaining appropriate weight, are healthy, or received the go-signal of your obstetrician, you can set your eating window for up to twelve hours every day.

While it is quite long to fall into the usual guidelines followed by various IF techniques, you can still expect this eating window to provide metabolic benefits. Another thing that you can do is to try promoting a balanced blood sugar level and healthy metabolism by ditching late-night snacks and focusing more on morning meals.

Doing so can help prevent certain complications such as gestational diabetes. To avoid gaining too much weight, you may want to stick to the rule of eating a healthy breakfast and preventing yourself from putting anything on your mouth after eight in the evening.

You can also improve your health while pregnant by increasing your consumption of fruits, nuts, and veggies. You have to get rid of processed foods and refined sugars from your diet, too. With that, you can have a healthy pregnancy without gaining too much weight even if you do not strictly adhere to IF rules.

Chapter 8 - Intermittent Fasting and Fertility: Does IF Help in Getting Pregnant?

If you are not pregnant yet but want to have a baby, then be aware that intermittent fasting can help in several circumstances. It is because of the mutually beneficial connection between fertility and diet. If you are either obese or overweight, have problems ovulating, or experience irregular cycles that tend to affect your fertility, then IF can help.

Note that following an IF diet means that you can lessen your calorie consumption with the limited eating window and scheduled fasting periods. This protocol can lead to weight loss, which can improve your fertility. Intermittent fasting can also help you deal with those issues that tend to cause difficulties in getting pregnant.

Intermittent fasting is also a big help for those women with fertility issues because of PCOS (polycystic ovary syndrome). It can specifically help those diagnosed with PCOS and obesity because fasting regularly can raise the level of luteinizing hormone in their bodies. Such an increase can contribute to more regular ovulation.

It has also been discovered that losing around five to ten percent of weight because of intermittent fasting can help a woman's reproductive system. Combined with IF's ability to deal with insulin resistance and other possible health concerns, your improved reproduction caused by fasting can improve your overall fertility. It also ensures that your reproductive system will continue to stay healthy.

Aside from that, intermittent fasting is known to regulate your hormones. It can improve your fertility if you are dealing with hormone-related issues that lead to infertility. However, you also have to be extra careful when implementing the IF approach to improve your fertility. Make sure to avoid being too intense when implementing it as it might only cause stress and pressure to your body.

If you do IF too aggressively, then it can stress your body, leading to infertility, instead. When trying to adhere to IF for fertility reasons, make sure to observe your cycle. Find out if you experienced changes in your cycle. If you notice some changes, then there is a high chance that your IF plan is too intense or aggressive.

In such a case, you have to consider scaling back your daily fasting window. Do so until you have discovered the right one for you. Some women find it more beneficial to stick to the 16:8 IF method, which is composed of a 16-hour fasting period and an 8-hour eating window. However, if you are new to it, it is advisable to start more slowly. For instance, you may want to start with an eating window of 10 hours then gradually reduce it to 8 hours.

Another thing to note is that this approach is not suitable for those who are underweight if the goal is to get pregnant. It is because restricting your food intake to a certain eating window and limiting your intake of calories can only hamper your fertility if your weight is lower than what is appropriate for you. There are even extreme cases wherein weight loss and IF can adversely impact fertility, especially if it results in stopping ovulation and menstruation.

If your goal is to get pregnant, then you can maximize IF's effects with the following tips:

- **Include eggs in your diet** – Make sure to include an egg in any of your meals during your eating window. Even just one egg is rich in nutrients that can nourish your egg cells. Eggs are rich in good fats and protein that can benefit your egg cells, especially if you eat them for breakfast.

- **Add pureed soups and broths into your diet** – The good news is that you can now find bone broth being conveniently packed and sold in health food markets. What is great about broths is that they are rich in dense nutrients. They can help nourish your bodies without significantly increasing your calorie intake, making them great to consume during your eating window.

  You may also want to enjoy pureed veggie soups composed of asparagus and zucchini. These soups are not only delicious but are also very filling. You can consume them at room temperature, promoting convenience. These soups also tend to work great during your period's cleansing week.

Just make sure that you do not end up replacing full meals with broths or soups only. A wise tip is to add it into a well-balanced diet, so you can supply your body with more nutrients.

- **Use coconut water for hydration** – You can also hydrate by drinking coconut water. It is a great way to replenish the lost fluids within your body. One thing to take note of is that your ovarian follicles have high levels of fluid, which is why you can also boost your fertility by staying hydrated.

  With the high electrolyte content of coconut water, you can achieve such hydration. Coconut water also has isotonic properties that resemble cellular fluid. These properties and components in coconut water can make you more fertile, so making them a part of your IF diet may help you get pregnant.

- **Modify your intermittent fasting routines** – You should also try modifying the IF approach you decided to follow depending on your current needs and requirements. For instance, if the fertility medication you are taking causes you to gain excess weight, causing more frustration, then you may want to modify your eating pattern.

  You can schedule your dinner early – around 7 in the evening, then have a nourishing breakfast before 8 in the morning. This the time when you have a high level of digestive enzymes. By ensuring that your breakfast consists of foods with proper nourishment, you will feel a lot better. This is also the key to the even distribution and assimilation of nutrients from the foods you eat. It is a big help in making you more fertile.

Aside from the mentioned tips, it is also highly advisable to avoid fasting for more than sixteen hours if your goal is to get pregnant. A fasting period of 16 hours or less is usually the most beneficial for those who want to improve their fertility.

Chapter 9 – Intermittent Fasting and Menstruation: Does IF Affect your Cycle?

With the continuous popularity of intermittent fasting, a lot of women who make IF a part of their regular diet also start wondering if constant fasting has an effect on their hormones, as well as their menstrual cycle. A lot of women experience things, like anxiety, sluggishness, and feeling off during their period.

You may experience these symptoms because of your hormones. Note that your hormones play a major role in how your body responds to specific eating plans. While intermittent fasting provides several benefits, there is still a time when you should not fast – that is usually a week or so before your menstrual period.

Remember that certain factors like your present weight, level of exercise, and caloric intake have an impact on the cycle of your reproductive hormones. For example, intense calorie restrictions, nutritional deficiencies, exercises, and weight loss can lead to amenorrhea or skipped or irregular periods.

When implementing intermittent fasting, you may not be able to get sufficient calories to support your reproductive health, leading to irregular menses. It may cause you to be unable to receive an adequate supply of metabolic or nutritional energy that can support pregnancy, which might signal your brain to stop its reproductive cycle. It is the reason why you have to be wary of fasting when your period is coming close.

IF and a Woman's Hormones

Just like what has been mentioned in several parts of this book, IF can be linked to several health benefits. However, it also seems to disrupt women's hormones. It can also trigger hormonal imbalances. It might disrupt the balance of your estrogen.

The problem with having an imbalanced estrogen is that it can have a few negative effects, like low energy, weight gain, inability to properly control your glucose, reduced bone density, and poor muscle tone. It might also impair your cognitive function and the health of your hair and skin.

Aside from that, you have to remember that even with only a single hormonal system being disrupted in the body, it can still cause other problems related to hormonal imbalance. Other major considerations regarding women's hormones, especially for those who follow IF, are thyroid hormones and cortisol, which is a stress hormone.

If your cortisol goes out of balance, it can lead to unwanted symptoms like lack of energy, insomnia, anxiety, excessive tiredness, and sugar cravings. If your thyroid hormones are the ones that go out of balance, then expect to experience weight gain, depression, anxiety, brain fog, dry skin and hair, inability to regulate body temperature, and irregular periods.

These negative effects of hormonal imbalance that might be triggered by intermittent fasting, especially during those times when your monthly period comes close, are among the major reasons why you have to practice this eating pattern correctly and safely. If you truly want to stick to this habit every day, then you have to constantly remind yourself that it is kind of tricky for women, so you have to try mastering it as much as possible.

Also, remember that your reproductive function has an intricate relationship with your metabolic function. With that in mind, if your body picks up signs of starvation from the environment, such as not feeding it for a long time, then it will most likely go into a mode where it preserves and protects.

When in that mode, your body will most likely hold onto weight as a means of surviving hunger, stimulate hunger hormone production so you will rush on finding food as soon as possible, and slow down bodily functions considered as non-essential, such as reproduction since doing so will prevent you from wasting energy on helping a baby grow and focus more on surviving.

However, it does not necessarily mean that you should stop IF altogether even if your body can handle it. This approach still carries plenty of benefits and missing even just a day might prevent you from enjoying such benefits.

With that said, it is advisable to learn and apply simple rules that will let you practice IF safely without significantly disrupting your menstrual cycle – one such rule is not fasting or just shortening your fasting period about a week before your actual period.

Why Fasting Should be Avoided a Week Before Your Period?

One thing you have to know about your menstrual cycle is that your body is more prone to dealing with stress around a week before your actual period. It is the time when you will have an extremely low level of estrogen. This can result in sensitivity to cortisol, a stress hormone.

It is the main reason why before your period, you will most likely notice major changes in your energy and mood. There are even instances when you experience extreme cravings for sugary stuff. Due to your body's sensitivity to stress during such time of the month, it is advisable to stay away from anything that might stress you out even further.

Some possible stressors are extreme workouts, intense diet plans, and intermittent fasting. While these stressors are beneficial since they can help improve your body's resilience and strength, it is still advisable to slow down during the times when your body is extremely sensitive to stress.

This means that one week before your period should be the time when you should let your body have a bit of rest. You do not want to stress your body more when you already feel naturally down because of your hormones. Try to consider this week as a time to give yourself proper care. Use this time to get a massage or do more self-care routines.

What Can You Do a Month Before Your Period?

While it is not advisable to fast when your period is nearing, it is still undeniable that fasting is a vital routine for a lot of women. With that in mind, there are those who may not like the idea of having to do a complete change in their habit a week or so every month.

If you are an avid follower of intermittent fasting and you feel like you will have a hard time breaking away from the habit, then you may want to reduce the number of hours you spend time on fasting. It is the best solution if you feel like you can't completely take a break from IF.

For instance, if you are following the 16:8 IF method, then you can reduce your fasting hours into 12 instead of the usual 18. Your goal should be to cut it down a bit to prevent your body from experiencing excessive stress.

Another tip is to take a magnesium supplement a week or so before your period. This can contribute to easing your PMS (premenstrual) symptoms. In case you are deficient in magnesium, include nuts and seeds rich in magnesium into your diet.

Is it Safe to Do IF on your Period?

Most recommendations when it comes to intermittent fasting as it relates to your menstrual cycle include avoiding fasting or trying to reduce the number of hours you fast only a week before your period starts.

This means that you can fast during your actual period. However, you have to prioritize your safety.

Practice intermittent fasting only after you have mastered how you can do it safely during your period. Here are some tips that can help you get through your period without having to stray away from your IF lifestyle:

- **Avoid jumping into intense fasting at the start of your period** – Once you have completed your self-care week, the time before your period, you may feel like it is time for you to begin fasting again. However, try not to jump into intense fasting right after your period begins. It would be best to do it around the second or third day of your period.

  Note that it is common for you to still experience some unwanted symptoms of menstruation, like tiredness, during the first day of your period. It is because it is usually the time when you have the heaviest flow. It is also the time when your body still tries to recover from the crash of your hormones.

  After around a couple of days, the level of your hormones will begin to rise, so expect to have more energy and feel a lot better. It is, therefore, the perfect time for you to kick up your workouts and fasting routines.

- **Shorten your fasting hours** – If you are used to fasting for long periods, then you should try making adjustments to it when your period is approaching as well as when it comes. As much as possible, fast only for less than twelve to thirteen hours. Avoid going longer than that period during your menstruation as it might only have negative effects on your hormones.

- **Avoid intense and extreme workouts during your fasting hours** – If you have the habit of working out, then avoid scheduling your workouts at your scheduled fasting periods. This tip is even more important during your actual period or a week before it.

  It is because intense exercises may stress out your body. Combine that with the kind of stress that fasting might also cause and your hormones will most likely be thrown out of balance.

- **Supply your body with nutrients for hormonal health** – During your eating window, do not forget to provide your body with the support it needs by supplying it with nutrients designed to improve your hormonal health. Eat healthy foods, particularly those that will prevent your hormones from going out of balance.

Aside from the mentioned tips, it also helps to observe your own body and its reactions to IF as soon as you start implementing it. If you notice that there are no major effects on your body and health even if you fast for a shorter period during your period and a week before it, then you may be able to increase your fasting period to a max of 16 hours.

However, do so gradually, and only after you have confirmed that fasting is something that your body can safely handle. Also, make sure that you constantly observe how you feel. Keep track of everything that you feel and reduce your fasting window or stop this habit completely just in case you experience severe signs of hormonal imbalance.

Among the hormonal imbalance symptoms you have to watch out for are:

- Sudden irregularity of your period – There are also instances when it stops completely.

- Sleeping difficulties

- Noticeable changes in digestion and metabolism

- Negative changes in your mood

- Brain fog

- Feeling cold all the time

- Negative changes on the look of your skin and hair

- Sudden inability to recover from workouts quickly and easily

- Slow healing from injuries

- Reduced tolerance to stress

It is also a must for you to keep track of and fully understand your reproductive cycle. It is the key to becoming one of the healthiest female intermittent fasters out there. To help you, you can use a period and reproductive health tracking app to give you an idea of your reproductive health.

With the help of such trackers, you can immediately sense if there is something that is not part of your usual pattern. If that is the case, then you can contact your doctor. You also need to monitor anything that disrupts your menstrual cycle. By gathering such information, you can better decide whether it would be more beneficial for you to lessen the number of days or hours you fast every month.

Your goal here is to get an idea about the specific way through which your body works. By knowing that, it will be easier for you to formulate decisions and make choices that are good for your hormones and reproductive health.

Make sure to listen to your body, too. If fasting seems to make you feel good and great, then continue doing it. However, if you notice some unwanted symptoms, having your hormones checked is a must.

That way, you will know if intermittent fasting works in your favor or not. If it does not, then you may want to take a break from the fast for a while to yield more favorable results as far as your hormones and overall health are concerned.

Chapter 10 – Intermittent Fasting and Aging: How Women Over 50 can Practice IF?

Intermittent fasting also seems to win the hearts of aging women, particularly those who are over 50. It is mainly because most of them noticed how good intermittent fasting is when it comes to helping them handle the aging process more efficiently.

One advantage of IF for women over 50 is that it seems to help them heal various aspects of their life. It is a big help in healing not only physically but also mentally and emotionally. Some of them also noticed how great IF is when it comes to making them more comfortable with their own body and health.

It also allows them to formulate better food choices, especially because the habit makes them fully aware of what being hungry truly feels. With that, they have a lower chance of succumbing to cravings.

Benefits of IF for Women Over 50

If you are wondering if intermittent fasting is good for you once you reach 50 and above, then you will be glad to know that such an eating pattern can indeed offer wonderful benefits for your age. Note that as you age, you will also most likely deal with issues regarding your weight, belly fat, joint, muscle, and bone health, metabolic syndrome, depression, and mood.

Intermittent fasting seems to help you handle those issues well. Here are just some of the areas where IF can benefit you and other women who are over 50:

Helps in safe and healthy weight loss

Probably the most significant benefit that IF can offer is weight loss. The weight loss effect of this famous eating pattern can also be experienced even if you reach 50. The eating pattern can even help women over such age lose excess belly fats successfully.

With belly fat being a major concern for a lot of postmenopausal women for reasons related to health and appearance, it is no longer surprising why intermittent fasting continues to become popular among that age group. The good thing about reducing belly fat through IF is that it can also help you lessen your risk of suffering from metabolic syndrome.

It refers to a set of health issues that might increase your risk of dealing with diabetes and cardiovascular diseases. IF results to weight loss and the reduction of belly fat especially because this approach requires you to consume regular meals within just a shorter period, leaving you to feel full and satiated the entire day.

The feeling of fullness you will experience from your regular meals can prevent you from grabbing and taking in unhealthy snacks in between each meal. Once it is time to fast, you can expect your body to reach the fasted state, which tends to foster and stimulate fat burning.

This goes for around 8 to 12 hours from your last meal, which makes it possible for you to maximize its fat-burning effects. With that, you can lose weight without having to make drastic changes in the quantity and type of food you consume as well as the frequency and length of your exercises.

Women over 50 who stick to a well-planned IF protocol can expect to enjoy weight loss effects of around 1-2 lbs. per week. If you combine this approach with a proper exercise – one that works well for your age, then it would be possible for you to enjoy an increase of around 3-4 lbs. per week.

Slows down the process of aging

Intermittent fasting also continues to capture the interest of aging women because it has anti-aging effects. It is mainly because fasting tends to supercharge your metabolism. With that effect, your body will become more effective when it comes to burning calories and breaking down essential nutrients.

This can also result in the slowing down of DNA degradation, a common scenario once you age. Aside from that, it can accelerate the repair of DNA. All these effects of IF can lead to the slowing down of the aging process.

Another advantage of fasting regularly is that it can also increase the supply of antioxidants within your body. The presence of these antioxidants prevents the breakdown of cells that might happen because of the damaging free radicals.

Moreover, fasting prevents the development of chronic inflammation, which often happens as you age. It is good for aging women because it allows them to enjoy a much better quality of life. Some even say that IF serves as their fountain of youth with its anti-aging effects.

Improves the health of joints and muscles

Intermittent fasting is also good for aging women with the ability of the fasted state to aid in improving the health of their joints and muscles. This specific benefit is the main reason why low back pain and arthritic symptoms are not so common among women who practice IF.

Fasting also has positive effects on the manner through which the body performs the hormone production process that has an impact on bone minerals, such as phosphate and calcium. With that, it is no longer surprising to see fasting having a strong connection to better bone health.

Encourages cell repair

Intermittent fasting is also a big advantage for women over 50, especially if you consider how good it is in encouraging cell repair. Note that IF can help encourage your body to focus more on cell repair since it no longer has to prioritize food digestion. This means that it can focus more on cell repair. With that, it is also possible for fasting to be a great aid in repairing your body and allowing it to perform its functions properly.

Helps prevent insulin resistance

Another benefit of IF for aging women is its ability to help them avoid insulin resistance. Note that this condition often takes place if your blood sugar is constantly on a high level. This problem might cause your body to be unable to respond well to the sugar in your blood. It means that your body will not be able to break it down well.

By following the IF protocol, you can have full control of your blood sugar level. You can also prevent your blood sugar level from spiking up since IF can deal with factors that can trigger insulin resistance, such as excess body weight, obesity, poor diet, inactivity, and high blood pressure.

Promotes better mental and physical health

You will also be pleased to know that intermittent fasting supports better mental and physical health as you age. It is good for the brain. It lets your brain function better and improves your ability to focus more on certain tasks. The fact that it helps improve your focus and brain function can contribute a lot to completing a huge part of your daily workload.

Intermittent fasting may also prevent certain mental health problems, like those linked to depression and anxiety. It is mainly because it stimulates mental clarity. It can improve your self-esteem and mood and lower your risk of suffering from depression and anxiety.

It is also good for your physical health with its ability to increase your body's good cholesterol level and lower the bad ones. Aside from that, intermittent fasting can help improve the way you control your glucose, lessen fat deposits found in your liver, and keep your blood pressure low.

One more thing that fasting can do is improve the state of the gut microbiome, which refers to the bacteria in your stomach. This improvement can contribute to better mental and physical health. It can further help in improving the quality of your sleep as well as your memory and cognitive function.

IF Methods that Work Well for Women Over 50

For intermittent fasting to work in your favor, it is crucial to determine what specific method will work for you and your age. Most aging women tend to benefit more from the following IF methods, provided they follow the protocol and guidelines correctly.

- **12-hour fasting** – This method is ideal for beginners. If you choose the 12-hour fast, then note that it involves eating during the first twelve hours of your day then fasting for the remaining 12 hours. Most of those who follow this routine simply skip eating breakfast and start eating only during lunchtime.

  In case you are used to eating breakfast and have a hard time skipping it, then you may want to eat your dinner early and make sure you prevent yourself from grabbing any evening or midnight snack. A lot of women aged 50 and above tend to stick to the 12-hour intermittent fasting approach since they noticed that it is easier to commit to it.

- **16-hour fasting** – If you want better and faster results, then you may want to try out the IF approach, which consists of a fasting period of 16 hours. You will have an 8-hour eating window in this approach. Aging women also find this approach easy to commit to because they can easily schedule two meals and 1-2 snacks within the 8-hour eating window.

- **5:2 fasting** – This specific IF method is suitable for women over 50 who can't seem to handle restricted eating windows on a daily basis. It is because this method lets you eat as you normally would for five days per week. Fasting should be done 2 days a week that should be split up. This means that your fasting days should not be consecutive and you have to limit your calorie intake during those days to 500 to 600 calories.

These methods that have also been discussed in detail in one previous chapter of this book tend to provide the most favorable benefits to aging women. These IF protocols also seem to be the ones that most aging women can easily stick to.

How to Practice IF and Make it Work?

As you hit the 50-year mark, expect to experience some issues related to your health, like sleeping difficulties, slower metabolism, lower muscle mass, and painful joints. If those issues are bugging you, then it is possible for IF to do its wonders for you. This eating pattern is even a fantastic solution in warding off or lessening age-related health issues that might occur to you once you hit 50 and above.

The good thing about IF is that it also aids in maintaining a healthy weight. However, you have to make sure that you implement it correctly. Your success will fully depend on its correct implementation. You need to follow its guidelines to ensure that you get the results you want.

Here are some tips in practicing IF and make it work if you are already over 50.

- **Consider setting your fasting schedule overnight** – If you want to ease into fasting without having to feel uncomfortable changes in your previous eating patterns, then setting the number of hours you intend to fast overnight can help. You can go for at least 12 hours without food, so fasting overnight is surely a wise move.

  You just have to think about not eating anything after an early dinner. Your next meal should be a late breakfast or lunch. If you do not feel hungry upon waking up at all, then delaying your breakfast a bit longer is advisable. You can increase your fasting hours to 14 in such a case.

- **Eat breakfast that is easy to digest** – If your chosen eating window allows you to consume breakfast, then make sure to choose foods that you can easily digest. One great choice is a healthy smoothie, a soup, or anything that is naturally more liquid.

- **Pick an IF plan that is truly appropriate for you** – Ensure that you spend time assessing your current state of health and determine if your age fits the IF plan or approach that you have in mind. If you are a beginner in this approach, then you may find the 5:2 approach tricky since it involves restricting your calorie intake for a day.

  It would be best for you to begin with something that you can easily incorporate into your current lifestyle. For instance, you can choose the 16:8 diet since it is easier to schedule your eating windows and fasting periods through this approach. You should then consider progressing from there if you achieve favorable results.

- **Consult an expert** – Note that since you are already over 50, consulting an expert, like a dietician or doctor, is vital as doing so can help ensure that you will not compromise your health by sticking to intermittent fasting. You have to talk to a professional to determine if your chosen IF approach is safe for you.

  By working with a professional, one who understands what you are trying to achieve from IF, you can figure out how to make the method work in your favor. You will also receive help on what to eat and what to avoid.

Make it a point to do minor changes first. Though they produce smaller gains, minor changes are still better as you have an assurance that they will not harm your body. Most of these minor changes can also produce long-term benefits.

- **Stick to healthy foods** – Ensure that the meals you eat during your eating windows consist of the healthy stuff. You can begin with protein. Note that at the time when the fast is already at the fat-burning stage, your body will most likely break down protein as a source of energy if you do not eat enough protein during your eating window.

  That said, make sure that you consume more protein to prevent muscle breakdown or loss. If possible, include protein in every snack or meal. Among the protein-rich foods, you can eat are eggs, protein shakes, beef, fish, chicken, Greek yogurt, and plant-based proteins, like lentils and beans. Balance this with other foods rich in nutrients, like fruits and veggies, as well as healthy sources of carbs, like quinoa, whole-wheat bread, and brown rice.

- **Pair it with an exercise** – You also have a higher chance of maximizing the benefits of intermittent fasting if you pair it with exercises that are safe for women over 50 to do. Just make sure to schedule your workout or exercise close to the end of your scheduled fasting hours. Time your workout in a way that it ends at the time when your feeding or eating window is already close.

Aside from the mentioned tips, it is also a must to listen closely to what your body is telling you, especially during the long periods of fasting. Find out if you are experiencing most of the following after you have started implementing intermittent fasting:

- A feeling of being weaker than usual

- Reduced endurance

- The same workouts suddenly become harder to fulfill than before.

- Sudden poor quality of sleep

- Reduced focus and concentration

- Feeling anxious and depressed all of a sudden

- Memory loss

- Being constantly distracted by hunger

If you experience most of the ones mentioned, then intermittent fasting may not be the safest approach for your age. You will instantly know that IF is working favorably for you if it does not make you feel miserable at all.

It is also crucial to take into account your present health and if you are already dealing with certain ailments. For instance, if you are someone who has to take medications together with food to prevent stomach irritation or nausea, then fasting may not be suitable for you.

If you are already taking blood pressure or heart medications, then be extra careful as fasting might increase your likelihood of having sodium and potassium imbalances every time you fast. Moreover, IF may also put your health in danger if you are suffering from diabetes and has to eat certain foods on a schedule or take medications that have a great impact on your blood sugar level.

Spend time talking to your doctor if you are already dealing with some health-related concerns, especially those linked to age. If you really want to give it a try, then discuss with him your intention to modify the approach so it will be safer for you.

For instance, you may want to reduce your eating window gradually until your body eases to the new routine or get used to it. In case you get the go-signal, observe your body's reactions. If you do not experience any negative effects but instead got the health or weight results you prefer, then making IF a part of your routine is most likely good for you.

Just make sure you do not forget to take your needed medications on time. You do not have to worry about your medications breaking the fast since they won't. You can also enjoy calorie-free drinks, such as black coffee or water, as those will not break your fast.

Chapter 11 – Top 10 Mistakes to Avoid When Practicing IF for Women

Intermittent fasting is generally safe for a lot of women. However, you have to do it correctly if you want to achieve the kind of results you want. You have to learn more about IF before starting to prevent committing certain mistakes that might only lead to failure. Here are just some of the most commonly committed mistakes of women who tried intermittent fasting that may cause you to become unsuccessful:

#1 - Not doing enough preparation

One thing you should remember about intermittent fasting is that it tends to go against the eating patterns considered normal in society. If you implement IF every day, then you will most likely see yourself scheduling your meals at unusual times. For instance, you may have to set your breakfast at 11 in the morning, instead of earlier. You may also have to schedule your dinner at 4 or 5 pm.

You may find these unfamiliar and odd meal schedules challenging, especially if you have a standard 9 to 5 job. It is the main reason why you should not jump into IF unprepared. Prepare for the sudden changes in eating patterns. You have to be fully prepared, especially for your feeding window.

For instance, if you are used to eating breakfast at home, then consider packing and eating it at work.

Note that if you don't prepare for it, then you will be at risk of making poor food choices that may only prevent you from getting the results you want from IF.

#2 - Not supplying your body with enough calories

While it is true that IF is implemented by many as a way to lessen their intake of calories, it does not necessarily mean that you have to have excessive restrictions on your calorie intake. Extreme calorie restrictions might lead to negative consequences, especially in athletes who need to consider their level of activities when deciding on an IF protocol.

They have to make sure that they still get sufficient calories to support and improve their athletic performance, recovery, and muscle growth. In case you have a hard time taking in sufficient calories within the eating window that you have allotted, try extending it so your goals will be supported while also optimizing your health.

#3 - Starting the IF protocol drastically

This is one of the major mistakes you should avoid committing. It means immediately jumping into IF and making drastic changes without giving your body and yourself the chance to adjust. If you do that, you will end up producing disastrous results.

For instance, if you are used to eating six small meals or three meals of normal sizes every day, then avoid limiting the eating window to just 4 to 6 hours especially if you are still a beginner. Your body will have a hard time adjusting to this new routine if you immediately jump into it.

Make sure that you do the process slowly instead of rushing into it. If you choose to implement the 16/8 IF protocol, then you can set your fasting times slowly. Do it slowly until you can reach the 16-hour fasting period.

#4 - Picking the wrong plan

Another mistake you should not commit when planning to implement IF is not studying the different IF plans or protocols. It is because it might lead you to pick the wrong plan. Before starting to shop for the foods you can eat during your eating window, make sure that you already studied all your IF protocol options and figured out which one will most likely produce your desired results.

For example, if you go to the gym for six days every week without fail, then it may not be a good idea to choose that plan, which requires you to fast completely for two days weekly. Do not choose a plan blindly and without thinking about what works for you. Spend time analyzing your present lifestyle and your goals. After that, choose a plan that perfectly suits your schedule, lifestyle, and habits.

#5 - Overeating during the eating window

Overeating during your feeding window is a possible trap that might cause you to fail when implementing IF. It might happen if your chosen regimen is too restrictive – one involving long hours of fasting. In such a case, you are likely to go overboard once the eating window comes. This means you are prone to eating more than what you need.

Remember that one possible reason why you decide to give IF a try is that it reduces your eating window, which may also lead to you consuming or taking in fewer calories. However, if you feel like your chosen plan is too restrictive, maybe causing you to get physically and emotionally starved, it would be hard to control your urge to eat a lot during your feeding time. It is especially true if you feel deprived.

With that, there is a risk that you will still eat the same number of calories that you will most likely consume within your fasting window. If that happens, then your goal of losing weight may be harder to reach. If you are one of those who are prone to overeating, then carefully plan what you are going to eat once your fasting window ends.

As much as possible, avoid eating your usual consumption of up to 2,000 calories in your eating window. What you should do, instead, is to create an eating plan, which will let you take in between 1,200 to 1,500 calories. Also, remember that the number of meals you will be eating should be based on how long your fasting window is.

If you feel like you are constantly deprived, causing you to have a hard time preventing yourself from overeating, then maybe it is time to reconsider your current eating plan. Find out if it is indeed the appropriate IF protocol for you. You may want to modify it a bit or look for another IF method that is more suitable for you. Your goal is to implement a method that makes you happy and satisfied.

#6 - Eating the wrong foods

Another possible mistake that tends to go hand in hand with the risk of eating too much is taking in the wrong foods. If your eating window is around 8 hours and you focus on eating more sugary, fatty, and refined foods during that period, then you will most likely not feel good.

While IF does not pose too many restrictions on what you should eat once during your feeding window, it is still advisable to commit to eating the healthy stuff if you want to be able to enjoy your desired results. Focus on eating more healthy fats, legumes, lean protein, wholesome fruits and veggies, nuts, and unrefined grains. These foods should be the usual inclusions in your diet.

It also helps to apply some principles and tips linked to clean eating. One is to cook at home. Make sure that you make it a habit to eat at home instead of dining in restaurants too often. Spending time reading nutrition labels should also be one of the tips you have to apply. Familiarize yourself with some of the forbidden ingredients, such as modified palm oil and high-fructose corn syrup.

Another wise tip is to monitor your intake of sodium. Be extra cautious of foods that may have hidden sugar, too. Stay away from processed foods. When it is mealtime, make sure that your plate has a great balance of healthy fats, lean proteins, healthy carbs, and fibers. All these tips can assure you that your body will receive nothing but the healthiest foods that will support your IF journey.

#7 - **Not drinking enough**

This mistake may also be accompanied by another one, which involves consuming the wrong liquid. Note that proper hydration is always a vital component of any IF protocol. Keep in mind that during the fasting period, you will most likely drink less because you will not take in the water usually consumed together with your meals and snacks.

The problem with not supplying your body with enough water is that it can cause unwanted side effects, like intense hunger, muscle cramps, and headaches. To prevent dehydration, ensure that your body gets sufficient amounts of water. You can also drink water with a couple of tablespoons of ACV, which is known for curbing hunger.

Other liquids you can drink during your fasting window are black coffee, as well as green, oolong, herbal, or black tea. Also, note that while having proper hydration is a must when you are fasting, you have to remember that consuming the wrong liquids may also cause unsuccessful results. It is the reason why you have to make sure that what you are drinking will not break your fast.

As much as possible, stay away from liquids filled with protein during your fasting period. One example of such liquid is bone broth. Note that such liquids tend to stop autophagy, which refers to the cellular process involving the breakdown and recycling of damaged molecules. It is a process that you have to promote, not stop, every time you fast.

Avoid diet sodas, too. Note that even calorie-free beverages are still not good for you when you are fasting if those are full of sugar. It is because zero-calorie sweeteners can still affect the level of your insulin negatively. They tend to stimulate your appetite, making it harder to control your cravings.

To avoid making the mistake of not drinking sufficient amounts of water or drinking the wrong kind, it is advisable to keep track of your level of hydration. Fortunately, there are now apps that you can download to help you track it. By monitoring your intake of water, you can keep yourself accountable. You can also motivate yourself to stick to plain tea, black coffee, or water every time you fast.

#8 - Not doing any physical activities

Sticking to the IF protocol should not be an excuse for you not to work out. Note that being sedentary is one of the biggest mistakes you can commit while you are trying to get the best results from this eating pattern. You may feel like exercising during your fasting period is foreign, especially if you are used to consuming a pre-workout snack.

However, you have to constantly remind yourself that there is stored energy within your body fats that you can use even without food. Working out when doing IF is even a perfect scenario because your physical activities can help you in using up your stored fats.

Your workouts can also help increase your HGH (human growth hormone), which can also lead to muscle building.

Just make sure to consult your doctor first before doing any form of exercise when you are following the IF protocol. Generally, though, it is safe to exercise when sticking to such an eating pattern. You can also maximize the effects of your workouts by keeping in mind these tips:

- **Schedule workouts during your eating period** – Make sure that you also consume healthy carbs and lean protein thirty minutes after each session.

- **For intense exercises, schedule it during your feeding window, too** – Eat something before an intense session to ensure that there will always be available glycogen stores.

- **Pick a workout routine, which suits your chosen fasting method** – For instance, if you decide to follow that IF protocol that requires you to fast for 24 hours, then avoid pushing yourself too much by doing intense activities. Focus on mild workouts and save the intense ones on your feeding days.

- **Stay hydrated** – You should be well-hydrated not only when you are fasting but also when working out.

- **Listen to the signals sent by your body** – Do not ignore body cues or signals. If you experience things like lightheadedness or weakness, then taking a short break from your workout or ending the session is a wise move.

Apart from the mentioned tips, you may also want to do low-impact activities, such as walking. If your IF method requires you to fast overnight and you schedule your workouts in the morning, then make it a point to consume a meal rich in protein after your exercise. By doing that, you can improve your muscle-building activities.

#9 – Not syncing it with your present lifestyle

Another mistake you should avoid if you want to get the best results from IF is not making it suit your current lifestyle. Before deciding on an IF approach, make sure to spend time considering your present lifestyle. That way, you can choose an approach, which perfectly blends with it.

You do not have to force yourself to follow an IF approach, which requires you to fast for 20 hours and eat for only 4 hours if your present lifestyle would greatly benefit from having a feeding window that is longer than that. Forcing yourself to eat only for 4 hours might only result in failure and frustration.

You may want to increase your feeding time a bit, especially if you are one of those whose level of productivity is hampered without food in their bodies. If you find yourself less productive with minimal food, then it may not be a good idea for you to prolong your fasting period or set up your eating window at the wrong time.

To ensure that you pick an IF method that suits your lifestyle, make it a point to monitor your hunger patterns and your schedule first. It is a big help in figuring out the most suitable approach for your present lifestyle. It also helps to schedule your eating window in a way that you can begin eating early in the morning and start fasting early in the evening if your current lifestyle requires you to do so or you are fond of eating early during the day.

However, if you like to eat at night and you have no time cooking within the day, then you can benefit from scheduling a smaller eating window in the evening. Your goal should be to figure out the best plan for you based on your lifestyle and schedule. You can then craft a plan based on it. By doing that, you have a higher chance of adhering to such a plan and get your desired results.

#10 – Giving up right away

Remember that IF requires patience and discipline. You need to commit to this eating pattern if you want to produce the best results. Also, keep in mind that it usually takes some time before you get used to the habit. If you are used to eating frequent meals, then you will most likely notice the first 4 to 5 days being extremely difficult to handle.

It would be the adjustment period, so expect to feel hungry, lightheaded, or a bit fatigued. There are also instances when you experience headaches because of the new eating pattern. However, no matter how difficult the first few days are, do not allow yourself to give up right away. Remind yourself that soon, these initial feelings of discomfort will pass.

After the first week or so, you will notice your body starting to adapt to the new routine. Your feelings of hunger will diminish and you will begin noticing your energy and focus coming back. However, do not forget to be very observant of the cues sent by your body.

If after the first week you still do not feel good, then there is a great chance that you are rushing the process. It could also be that you picked the wrong plan for you. In that case, you may want to make adjustments or determine if another plan can make you feel better.

Other Points to Consider

Aside from avoiding the top 10 mistakes mentioned here, you also have to avoid pushing yourself too hard. For instance, you may extend your fasting period if you feel like your body can still handle it even if it already goes beyond the number of hours that your chosen method allows. Keep in mind that extending your fast will never supercharge the method's powers.

If you constantly feel the need to extend your fast even when not necessary, then consider talking to your doctor or a professional whose specialty is in eating disorders. You may not be suffering from an eating disorder but if food starts to make you feel regretful or remorseful, then having an expert by your side to guide you in the process can help.

Do not leave such negative feelings about food and your new eating pattern undealt with or untreated as it might only create bigger problems later on. Talk to a specialist to prevent it from turning into a full-blown eating disorder.

Chapter 12 – Additional Tips and Tricks to Get the Most Out of IF

Intermittent fasting can give you your desired results, especially in terms of losing weight and improving your overall health. To maximize its positive effects, here are some tips and tricks that will surely make you the most out of it.

Learn the difference between wanting and needing to eat

Before practicing IF, you have to make sure that you already know how to differentiate real hunger from just wanting to eat. It is because once you fast, you may have a difficult time controlling yourself whenever your stomach starts to growl. If you do not know how to differentiate real hunger, then it would be harder for you to get through the remaining hours of your fast.

To help you, you should tune in closely to the cue sent to you by hunger. Determine if it is actual hunger or if it is just brought by other feelings, like boredom. In case the hunger is caused by boredom, it would be best to look for a task that would distract you. For instance, you may start distracting yourself by cleaning up your inbox with unnecessary emails.

If you feel really hungry without experiencing some signs that you need to break the fast as soon as possible, like dizziness and weakness, then you can deal with it by sipping warm tea. A wise choice is peppermint tea since it is known to lessen appetite. You can also fill up your stomach by drinking a glass or two of water.

If you are practicing the IF protocol for quite a while now and you notice your body not adapting to it yet (could be because you still have feelings of extreme hunger especially during your fasting period), then think carefully about what you can do to handle the eating pattern more effectively. One thing that you can do is to incorporate a more calorie-dense or nutrient-dense food during your eating window.

You should also reflect on whether or not the plan is a suitable choice for you. If not, consider your present lifestyle, your health condition, your schedule, and your goals to figure out another IF plan that will work for you. You may also want to modify your current plan a bit.

Another tip is to include healthy fats, like avocado, olive and coconut oils, and nut butter into your diet plan. Include foods rich in lean protein, too. That way, you can satisfy yourself during the eating period and keep yourself full for longer, thereby preventing you from feeling extreme hunger once you begin to fast.

Do not make any exceptions for what you can take in outside your feeding window

Make sure that during your fasting period, you strictly follow what you are only allowed to consume. For instance, you should avoid taking in any food or drink that contains calories and energy. It is because it will only break a fast. In other words, you should not add butter or milk in your coffee nor take a glass or two of wine while you are still fasting.

Note that you can only consider the fast as real if you do not eat anything. This means there are no exceptions to what you are only allowed to consume. The only things that you should put in your body during that time would be water, black coffee, and herbal tea. Resist the temptation to drink sweetened beverages even if those were labeled as zero calories. It is because even if a sweetener does not contain calories, it can still cause an insulin response that may only ruin the benefits of IF.

Do not binge during your eating window

Do not use the long hours of not eating as an excuse to eat without control. Keep in mind that while some people greatly benefit from waiting for long periods to take all or most of their daily calorie needs, this habit can cause binge eating in others. It can result in some people taking in more foods than what your usual meals spread the entire day contain.

Binge eating or overeating is not also highly recommended during the evening. You should prevent yourself from overeating especially if your bedtime is already close since it might only lead to poor sleeping patterns. It can also disrupt your circadian rhythm. It may also cause you to wake up feeling bad about yourself.

This can undermine the supposed effect of IF, which is to make you feel better. To avoid binge eating, especially during the evening, make sure to shift the eating window to earlier hours. For instance, you can set it at 11 in the morning to 7 in the evening. That way, you have a lower chance of binging or overeating during late hours.

Do not beat yourself too hard

You can also gear yourself up for success if you do not beat yourself too hard in those instances when you slip out of your new eating pattern. Keep in mind that a single slip does not necessarily mean that you are already up for failure.

There will always be days when you feel like sticking to the IF regimen is extremely hard, causing you to slip up. If that happens, commit to not being too hard on yourself. Remind yourself that it is okay to give yourself a break from the habit. You can always give yourself some time to refocus – probably a day of not doing the regimen.

You may also stick to a healthy eating pattern but make sure to give yourself treats every once in a while. Do not let IF consume your entire life. It should just be a part of a healthy habit and lifestyle. You should still let yourself enjoy, spend time with loved ones, and work out.

Monitor your meals

You also have to keep track of the foods you eat to increase your chances of achieving success. Even if you set up everything correctly, not monitoring the foods you eat during your eating window will still cause you to fail. Also, remember that even if intermittent fasting is an effective tool for weight loss, you still need to adhere to the guidelines linked to energy balance.

What it means is that you can only achieve your goal of losing weight if you take in fewer calories than what is burned by your body. For instance, if your body burns up to 2,000 calories daily, then it is necessary to eat less than 2,000 calories every day to get rid of your excess weight. This principle is applicable whether you implement fasting or not.

Avoid perceiving IF as a magical solution to weight loss that still gives you the freedom to consume all the foods you want. If you have that mindset, then you will be unable to have any progress. Before starting your IF journey, make sure that you are already aware of the number of calories you should be consuming.

If possible, use apps that can help you monitor your meals. With that, it would be easier for you to guarantee a calorie deficit that will let you produce favorable weight loss results quickly.

Avoid eating too little

Yes, you need to limit your intake of foods during your eating window, especially if your goal for practicing IF is to lose weight. However, you have to be extra careful that you do not end up taking in only too little calories. Note that fasting may have an impact on the hormones regulating your appetite.

This might cause you to be unable to feel hunger for much longer than usual if your body has already adapted to the routine. It may also cause you to feel full right away even by just eating a small amount during your eating window. The problem is not getting enough calories can also cause problems to your body.

If your calorie intake is insufficient, then you are at a higher risk of losing too much energy. This might affect your work performance and your daily routines. If that happens, then you may also end up skipping the fasting routine every now and then.

Break the fast if it is necessary

This means that you should eat if you feel like it is necessary for your safety. Technically, extreme fatigue and hunger do not usually occur when fasting, especially if you adhere to the 16:8 method. However, you still have to observe your body and the signals it tends to send out.

For instance, if you feel extreme lightheadedness, then it might be because your body is sending you some signal. It could be that your blood sugar level has dipped too low, causing the need to eat something. In that case, do not feel guilty. It is always okay to break the fast whenever a certain situation calls for it.

Make wise food choices every time you need to break a fast. A wise tip is to grab a snack rich in protein, such as some turkey breast slices. You may also reach out for a couple of hard-boiled eggs. This will let you healthily break your fast. Go back to fasting if you feel like you have already returned to normal.

Other Intermittent Fasting Do's and Don'ts for Women

- **Avoid 24-hour fasts as much as possible** – Fasting for 24 hours or more is not that highly recommended for women, so try to avoid it as much as possible. It is because this routine may only increase your risk of being too weak and hungry, leading to increased intake of food and eventually weight gain. However, if you think your body can handle the 24-hour fasts, then do not stop yourself from doing so. Just make sure that it is truly healthy and safe for you.

- **Rest and relax every once in a while** – During your fasting window, avoid doing extremely strenuous exercises. Stick to light exercises, like yoga. Make sure to do some activities that will let you rest and relax, too. Your goal is to enjoy your IF journey instead of stressing yourself out over minor mistakes or slip-ups.

- **Make each calorie count** – If you choose an IF plan that lets you eat some calories even if you are fasting, then ensure that each calorie that you take in counts. Pick nutrient-dense foods, particularly those with high fiber, healthy fat, and protein content. Some examples are eggs, avocado, nuts, fish, beans, and lentils.

- **Improve the taste of your foods without increasing calories** – For instance, you should season your meals with herbs, vinegar, spices, or garlic. These ingredients have extremely low-calorie content but are capable of significantly improving the flavor of your foods.

- **Do not obsess over food** – Instead of obsessing over the foods you can eat during your eating window, set up some distractions, especially during the times when you need to fast. You should be able to distract yourself, so you won't think too much about foods that may only lead to overeating or binge eating. Some distractive activities are watching a movie and finishing up some paperwork.

- **Do not fast if you do not feel well** – Keep in mind that while fasting can cause a few discomforts, like the feeling of irritability, hunger, and tiredness, it should never cause you to feel unwell. If you feel ill, stop the fast and contact your doctor right away. Among the signs of being unwell that you have to watch out for are extreme weakness and tiredness that make it hard for you to do your tasks.

Follow the tips and tricks mentioned in this chapter and you will surely have a better chance of achieving the results you are hoping for from intermittent fasting.

Chapter 13 – Frequently Asked Questions About IF for Women

Is intermittent fasting difficult to adhere to?

It could be difficult for some people. You may experience difficulties and challenges especially if you are still a beginner and your body still adjusts and adapts to the new routine and pattern of food intake. Once your body adapts, you will find the eating pattern more manageable and easier to follow.

The main premise is being more aware of when and what you should eat. With such awareness, you will know exactly the boundaries and limitations you have to keep in mind. Also, it would be best to pair this approach with daily exercise and making healthy food choices, like fruits, beans, veggies, healthy fats, lean proteins, and lentils.

Avoiding too much sugar and sodium is a must, too. Once your body adapts to these new guidelines, adhering to IF will no longer be that challenging.

What is the recommended number of hours/days for fasting?

In most cases, followers of the IF approach set their fasting window to up to 16 hours daily. Most follow this routine as it is a bit easy to adapt and adhere to. You can do it just by skipping breakfast after you eat your last meal the other day. If you can, you may also practice the IF pattern, which requires you to go without food for 24 hours straight twice every week.

Do I still need to count calories?

The answer to this will depend on the goals you want to achieve while practicing IF. It is not necessary in some cases but if your goal is to lose weight, then you may want to still monitor your calorie intake.

Also, if you plan to cut out on snacks before sleeping or go without eating for a long period, then you will notice your calorie count declining naturally. Another thing to note is that taking in foods that are mostly plant-based will also naturally lower your calorie intake.

Should women do IF differently?

In most cases, men and women tend to respond differently to the IF protocol. Most women also agree that they tend to achieve better results by widening their eating window a bit. For instance, when trying to follow the 16/8 IF plan, some women noticed that they get better results after they modified the approach – that is increasing the number of eating hours to 10 and reducing the fasting hours to 14.

A wise advice is to experiment and find out which one works for you. Observe the signals and cues sent by your body. Determine how it reacts to a specific IF pattern, too. Make sure to stick to an approach that seems to stimulate positive and favorable responses from your body.

Is it safe for pregnant or breastfeeding women to fast?

Intermittent fasting is not highly recommended for pregnant women. It is mainly because your focus during pregnancy should be to supply your body with nutrients that can support your health and the growth and development of your baby. You need to eat highly nutritious foods that will help develop and build your baby's body and brains.

Also, take note that there are pregnant women who have a hard time having enough iron stores. If you do not eat the required foods every day, then it might lead to iron deficiency, which is important for your baby. Despite that, there is still no rule that bans pregnant women from practicing IF.

If you are one of those who have already practiced it and your health is at its best, then following IF is most likely safe for you. Just make sure that you only do it after receiving the consent from your doctor. Also, it would be best to shorten the fasting period. If you are used to doing it for 24 hours or more, then avoid doing it while you are pregnant. You should fast for at most 14 to 16 hours only.

If you are breastfeeding, long fasting periods also need to be avoided. It is because of the constant need of your baby for nutritional milk. Fasting may have a huge impact on the quality and production of breast milk so you have to be extra careful. A wise advice is to avoid fasting for more than 12 to 14 hours if you are breastfeeding to ensure that the production of milk will not be interrupted.

Make sure to observe yourself and the body, too. If you notice that your milk supply suddenly dries up and you suspect that it is because of IF, then stop fasting right away. Try to eat more regularly to find out if doing so resolves the issue. If you notice fasting greatly hampering your milk production, then maybe it is time to stop it for a while and just continue once you already stop breastfeeding.

Can I still work out even if I am doing IF?

Of course, you can. If your fasting period is 24 hours or more, then you may want to schedule your workouts during your non-fasting days to ensure that you have more energy to complete the sessions. You can also see other women working out even during their fasting periods, especially if their fasting takes less than 24 hours.

It is because they notice how effective exercising during a fast is in building lean muscle mass. In general, you should schedule your exercise based on how your body feels as well as the workout habits you are used to.

Conclusion

Intermittent fasting is indeed something that women should do to improve their health and fitness. However, before starting this eating pattern, it is crucial to understand how it works exactly. Gather as much information about this approach as possible, so you will be guided once you start making it a part of your routines.

Also, determine the specific reasons why you want to fast in the first place. It could be that you want to challenge yourself, put limitations on your eating window, lose weight, or begin adopting healthy habits. You have to know the exact reason why you want to do it as such will help you decide on the most suitable IF plan for you.

By knowing exactly the reason for adapting IF, you will have an easier time keeping track of your progress and evaluating its results. You will know right away if it is indeed working favorably for you and helping you meet your goals.

*****

Thanks for downloading my book. Make sure to leave a short review on Amazon if you like it. I'd like to read your opinion. This means a lot to me.

www.ingramcontent.com/pod-product-compliance
Lightning Source LLC
Chambersburg PA
CBHW070831260726
48654CB00025B/933